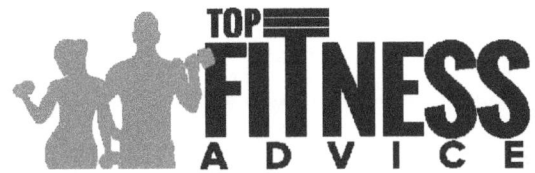

KETOGENIC DIET

79 Ketosis Recipes That Use Foods PROVEN To Fire Up Your Body's Fat Burning Potential (Breakfast, Lunch, Dinner & Snacks Included)

Kayla Bates

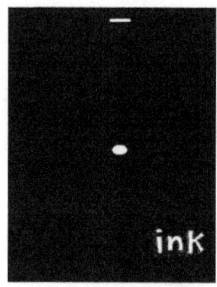

First published in 2017 by Venture Ink Publishing

Copyright © Top Fitness Advice 2019

All rights reserved.

No part of this book may be reproduced in any form without permission in writing from the author. No part of this publication may be reproduced or transmitted in any form or by any means, mechanic, electronic, photocopying, recording, by any storage or retrieval system, or transmitted by email without the permission in writing from the author and publisher.

Requests to the publisher for permission should be addressed to publishing@ventureink.co

For more information about the contents of this book or questions to the author, please contact Kayla Bates at kayla@topfitnessadvice.com

Disclaimer

This book provides wellness management information in an informative and educational manner only, with information that is general in nature and that is not specific to you, the reader. The contents of this book are intended to assist you and other readers in your personal wellness efforts. Consult your physician regarding the applicability of any information provided in this book to you.

Nothing in this book should be construed as personal advice or diagnosis, and must not be used in this manner. The information provided about conditions is general in nature. This information does not cover all possible uses, actions, precautions, side-effects, or interactions of medicines, or medical procedures. The information in this book should not be considered as complete and does not cover all diseases, ailments, physical conditions, or their treatment.

You should consult with your physician before beginning any exercise, weight loss, or health care program. This book should not be used in place of a call or visit to a competent health-care professional. You should consult a health care professional before adopting any of the suggestions in this book or before drawing inferences from it.

Any decision regarding treatment and medication for your condition should be made with the advice and consultation of a qualified health care professional. If you have, or suspect you have, a health-care problem, then you should immediately contact a qualified health care professional for treatment.

No Warranties: The author and publisher don't guarantee or warrant the quality, accuracy, completeness, timeliness, appropriateness or suitability of the information in this book, or of any product or services referenced in this book.

The information in this book is provided on an "as is" basis and the author and publisher make no representations or warranties of any kind with respect to this information. This book may contain inaccuracies, typographical errors, or other errors.

Liability Disclaimer: The publisher, author, and other parties involved in the creation, production, provision of information, or delivery of this book specifically disclaim any responsibility, and shall not be held liable for any damages, claims, injuries, losses, liabilities, costs, or obligations including any direct, indirect, special, incidental, or consequences damages (collectively known as "Damages") whatsoever and howsoever caused, arising out of, or in connection with the use or misuse of the site and the information contained within it, whether such Damages arise in contract, tort, negligence, equity, statute law, or by way of other legal theory.

Table of Contents

Disclaimer	3
Introduction	7
How to Use This Book	11
Chapter 1: Breakfast	15
Chapter 2: Lunch	43
Chapter 3: Dinner	83
Chapter 4: Snacks	147
Conclusion	163
Final Words	164

Would you prefer to listen to my book, rather than read it?

Download the audiobook version for free!

If you go to the special link below and sign up to Audible as a new customer, you can get the audiobook version of my book completely free.

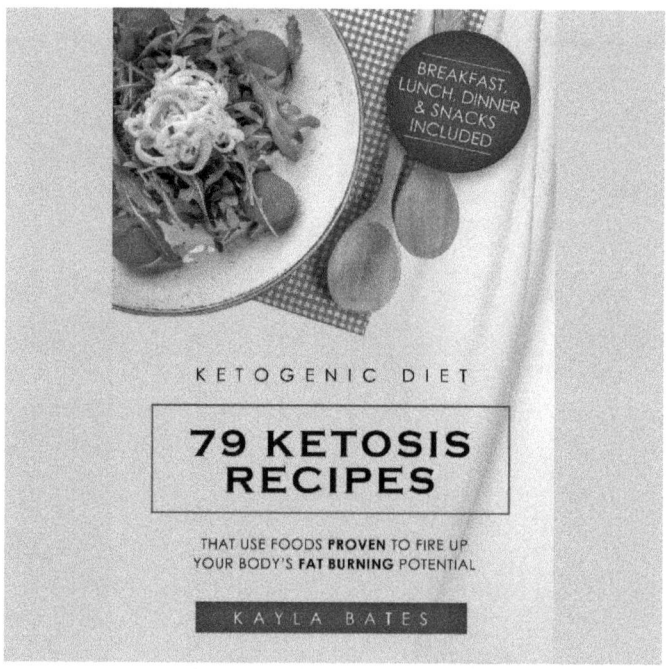

Go here to get your audiobook version for free:

TopFitnessAdvice.com/go/KetoDiet79

Introduction

When it comes to commonly held beliefs, most people have been told that eating too much fat is what makes us sick. Whilst it is true that eating too many calories in a day is bound to lead to weight gain, cutting out fat is also not the answer.

Fat came under fire because it is very calorie dense. It seems to make sense – cut out the more nutrient dense food in order to drop the number of calories that you consume.

However, if you consider that we evolved as hunter-gatherers who might have had to go without food for a day at a time or more, the picture becomes more complicated. Our bodies are not built for having such ready access to food in general and carbs in particular. Our ancestors had to go out and hunt for their food. Today though, we just stop in at the store.

Pair that with our increasingly sedentary lifestyles and it is hardly surprising that we are becoming more obese and that dieting is such a huge trend.

But, despite the fact that the typical low-fat diet has been punted as the best option for the last few decades, we are getting more obese. Despite us cutting out so much fat, we are increasingly unable to lose the weight.

But look for a minute at what it is that we do eat. We take the fat out of food and it no longer tastes so good so we add in tons of sugar. The typical Western diet consists of a high level of processed foods that are high in sugar.

However, these highly processed carbs have very little nutrient value and, because they are so processed, they have a massive impact on our blood sugar levels.

We eat the carbs and our blood sugar levels skyrocket. The body responds by increasing the production of insulin. The sugar is mopped up and your energy levels plummet again. You then crave even more carbs to fuel your body.

You quickly get caught in a vicious cycle – you need the carbs for energy but they cause your blood sugar levels to crash fairly quickly. And, after the crash, your body requires more energy and so you have to eat again.

If this happens over and over again, your body becomes less responsive to the insulin produced by it. You end up needing more insulin to clear out the excess blood sugar. More insulin is produced but it is less effective than before.

More of the glucose that is produced is left over in the blood stream and is converted to fat that gets stored in the body.

The way to get out of this cycle, is to fuel your body in a completely different way. That is where a ketogenic diet comes in to play.

Ketosis can reverse this by forcing your body to use the fat stores for energy.

The ketogenic diet turns our commonly held belief about weight-loss on its head. Instead of cutting out as much fat as possible, you eat a diet that is high in protein and that has moderate amounts of fat and that restricts carbs as much as possible.

With the lack of glucose as a fuel source in the diet, the body has no choice but to start burning through the fat stored in it. Your body actually changes its preferred fuel source over to fat – and that is why you need to increase the amount of fat that you eat.

The benefits of a ketogenic diet is that you will not feel hungry or deprived in any way and you will be able to lose weight easily. Once the initial adjustment period is over, you will find that you have a lot more energy and a greater ability to focus.

We are not going to go into the actual diet in full in this book but we do provide you with recipes that are all keto-friendly.

Good luck!

How to Use This Book

Choose one breakfast, one lunch, one dinner and either one or two snacks a day and you will start to feel the benefits for yourself.

Unless otherwise stated, the following will apply to all recipes:

- All temperatures are in Fahrenheit.

- Do no use foods that are sweetened already – if necessary, the recipe will list what sweetener to use.

- Use organic, naturally produced food wherever possible.

Are You ALWAYS Hungry When You Try to Lose Weight?

Discover How to STOP Starving Yourself & Lose Weight FASTER By Eating MORE Food!

For this month only, you can get Kayla's best-selling & most popular book absolutely free – *The Ultimate Guide to Healthy Eating & Losing Weight Without Starving Yourself!*

Get Your FREE Copy Here:
TopFitnessAdvice.com/Book

Discover how you can **start eating MORE food** and see weight loss results faster than ever before. Learn about the 10 most powerful fat-burning foods and how they boost the rate that your body burns fat. And last but not least, finally put an end to your emotional or "bored" eating habits. With this book, readers were able to significantly improve their weight loss results. So, it's highly recommended that you get this book, especially while it's free!

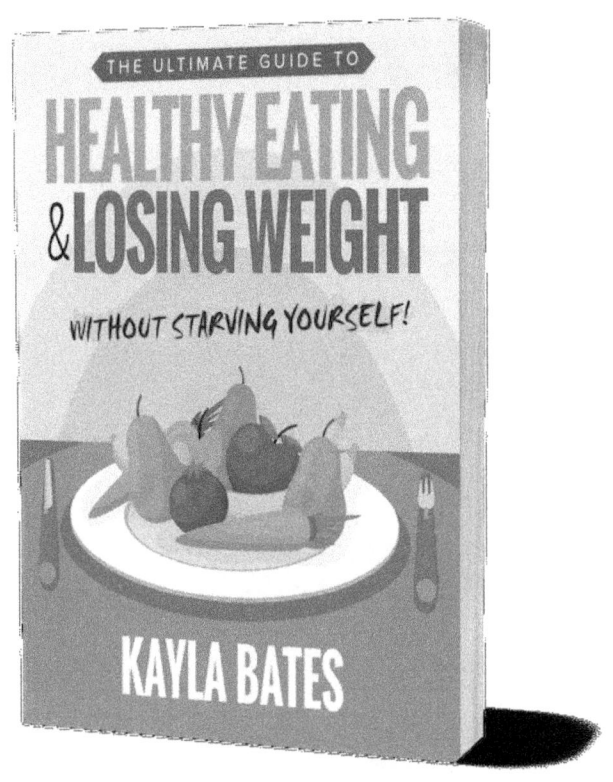

Get Your FREE Copy Here:

TopFitnessAdvice.com/Book

Chapter 1

Breakfast

1. Sage and Pork Patties

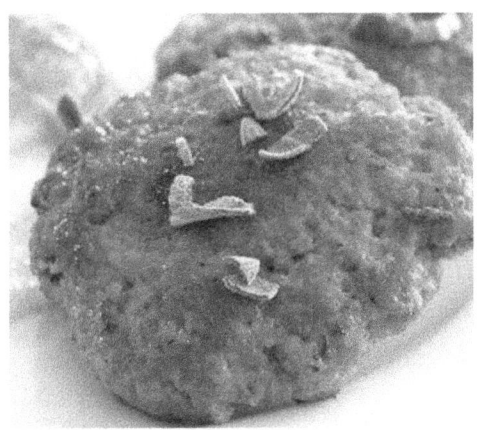

Serves 4

Ingredients

- 2 tablespoon fresh sage, chopped
- 1 pound ground pork
- 2 tablespoon Sweetener of your choice
- 1 teaspoon salt
- 1 teaspoon maple extract
- ½ teaspoon pepper
- ⅛ teaspoon cayenne pepper
- ¼ teaspoon garlic powder

Method

Mix together all the ingredients until completely mixed. Divide into eight evenly-sized balls and flatten into patties that are about an inch thick. Set your over to Medium and melt some farm butter or oil. Fry the patties for about four minutes on each side or until done.

2. Eggs Benedict

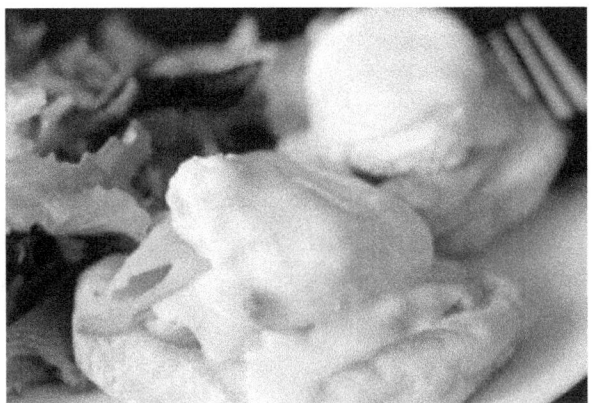

Serves 6

Ingredients for Bun

- ½ teaspoon fresh dill
- ¼ cup or whey protein
- 3 eggs, separated

Ingredients for Hollandaise Sauce

- ¼ cup lemon juice
- 6 large egg yolks
- 2 tablespoons Dijon mustard
- Seasoning to taste
- 1½ cups melted farm butter

Additions

- 12 large eggs

- 6 slices of prosciutto or ham

Method

Making the Buns: Set your oven at 325. Whip up the egg whites until they are really stiff. Fold in the whey powder and dill. Then fold in the yolks. Grease a baking tin and divide the dough evenly into buns about the size of a burger bun. Bake until they are nice and golden. (About twenty to thirty minutes.) Set aside to cool completely.

The Hollandaise Sauce: Set your stove to High and place a double boiler to heat up. Whisk together the lemon juice, mustard powder and yolks until combined. Put in the double boiler and whisk while adding in the butter. Cook until it starts to thicken, whisking all the while. Season to taste and whisk until thick – it will take a few minutes. Take off the heat and put to the side.

Assembly: Halve the buns and put a piece of prosciutto or ham on top. In the meantime, poach the eggs till they are done to your liking and put onto the bun. Add two or three tablespoons of the sauce to each bun.

3. Salmon and Avocado

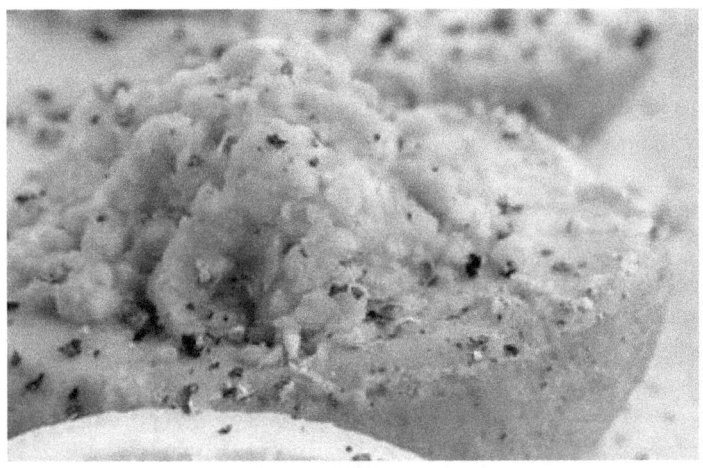

Serves 2

Ingredients

- 2 ounces of smoked salmon
- 1 large avocado
- 1 ounces of mild-flavored goat cheese
- a pinch of table salt
- the juice of 1 lemon
- 2 tablespoons of extra virgin olive oil

Method

Halve the avocado in two and take out the pit. Mix everything else in a blender or processor until chopped coarsely. Spoon into the avocado.

4. Ricotta and Chard Pie

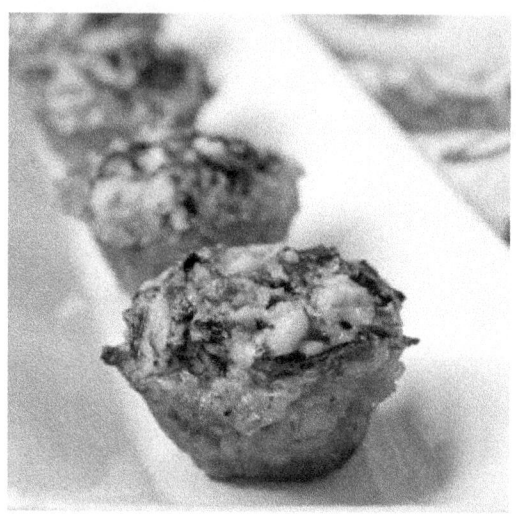

Serves 4

Ingredients

- ½ cup onion, coarsely chopped
- 1 Tablespoon olive oil
- 1 clove of crushed garlic
- 2 cups ricotta cheese
- 8 cups swiss chard, chopped up nice and finely
- 3 eggs
- ¼ cup fresh parmesan, grated
- 1 cup mozzarella, grated
- ⅛ teaspoon powdered nutmeg
- 1 pound pork sausage
- Seasoning to taste

Method

Set the stove to Med-High and heat up a big frying pan. Warm up the olive oil and then add in the garlic and onions. Fry until softened and then add the swiss chard. Cook for a few minutes until the leaves have just wilted. Season to taste and add in the nutmeg. Take off the heat and let it cool. In a clean bowl, whisk together the eggs and cheeses. Add the cooled greens.

Set your oven to 350. Remove the casing of the sausages and press it out into a greased pie plate until the base is covered. Add the filling on top and put on a baking sheet into the over. Bake for about half an hour till it firms up. You can alternatively divide the mixture amongst muffin tins. Just don't fill them more than three quarters full.

5. Quick Fix Eggs

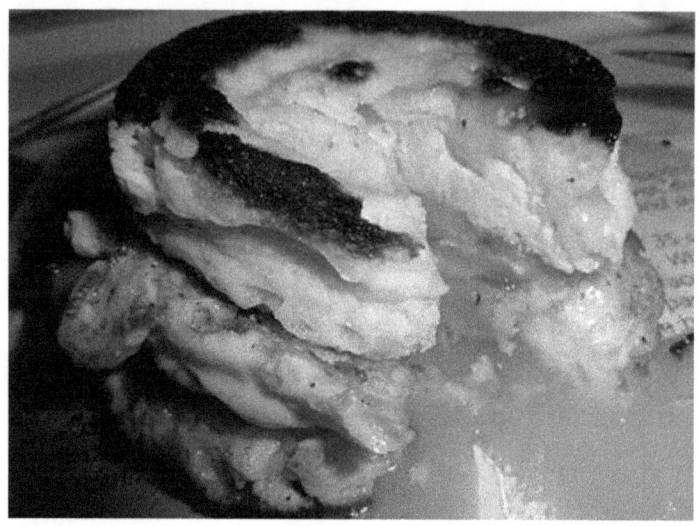

Serves 1

Ingredients

- 2 tablespoons fresh Parmesan, grated
- 1 ounce cream cheese, softened
- 1/2 teaspoon psyllium husks
- 1/2 teaspoon apple cider vinegar
- 1/8 teaspoon baking powder
- Garlic flakes to taste
- Seasoning to taste
- 2 large eggs, 1 of which should be separated
- 1/2 slice cheese
- 2 tablespoons olive oil, divided

Method

Cream the cream cheese, baking powder, Parmesan, vinegar, Psyllium husks, egg white and seasoning. Divide a tablespoon of the olive oil evenly between two ramekins and add the batter. Microwave on high for 30-45 seconds or until firm. Set your stove to Medium and coat the base of a frying pan with half of the rest of the olive oil.

Take the "biscuits" out of the ramekins and fry until lightly browned on both sides. Place the cheese slice on one biscuit while the biscuits are still warm. Place the rest of the oil into your frying pan. Crack the remaining egg along with the leftover yolk. Fry until done to your liking and put onto the biscuit. Top with the remaining bun and serve.

6. Sausage and Cheese Biscuits

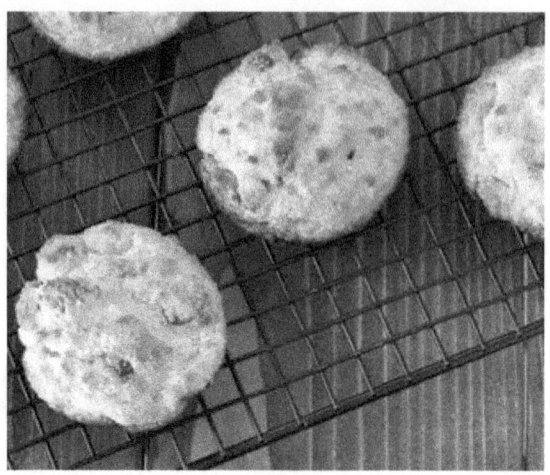

Makes 8

Ingredients

- 1 large egg
- 4 ounces of soft cream cheese
- 2 crushed cloves of garlic
- 1/2 teaspoon table salt
- 1 tablespoon chive, snipped
- 1/2 teaspoon Italian seasoning
- 1 cup mature cheddar, grated
- 1 1/2 cups almond flour
- 1/4 cup heavy cream
- 6 ounces of sausage meat, cooked – place on a paper towel once cooked to get as much of the grease off as possible
- 1/4 cup of plain water

Method

Set your oven at 350. Briskly whisk the egg and cream cheese. Add the seasonings, chives and garlic. Blend with the cream cheese. Add the water, flour, cheese and cream. Mix very well. Fold the sausage meat in and grease the wells of a muffin tin. You will only need 8 of the wells. Divide the dough between the different wells and then bake for 20-25 minutes. Allow the muffins to cool completely before you try to take them out.

7. Frittata's with A Kick

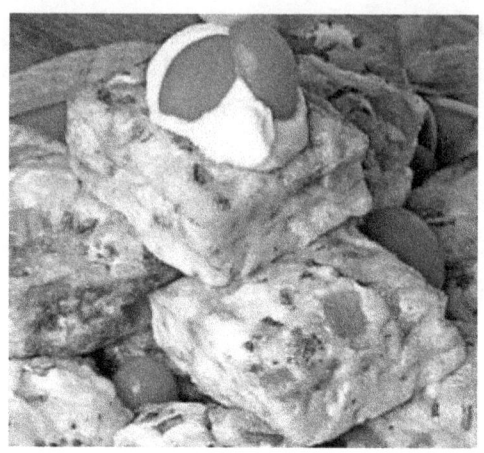

Serves 12

Ingredients

- 2 cups mild bell peppers
- 8 ounces pork sausage meat
- 10 eggs
- 2 egg whites
- 1/2 cup milk
- 1/2 teaspoon table salt
- 1/2 cup pepper jack
- 1/4 teaspoon pepper
- Toppings: Spring onion, sour cream, salsa and cilantro

Method

Set oven to 350. Set your stove to Med-High and fry the met till done. Take it out with a slotted spoon and put to one side. In the pan juices, fry up the peppers until they start to soften. In a clean bowl, mix together the milk, the egg whites and eggs.

Grease a 12-well muffin pan and divide the cooked sausage and peppers evenly between each and do the same with the egg mix. Divide the cheese in the same way and stir it up. Bake for about half an hour or until done through and slightly golden.

8. Breakfast Squash

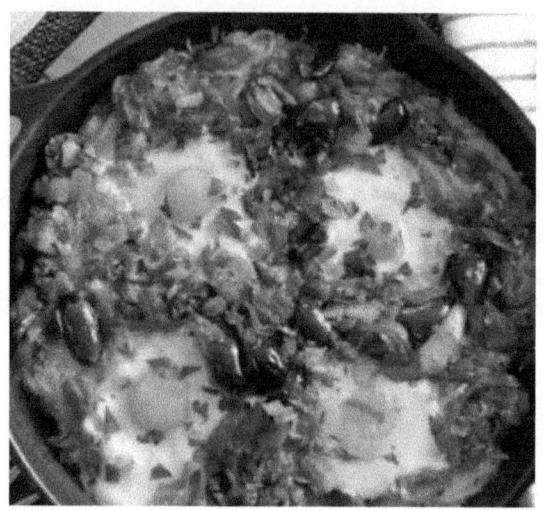

Serves 4

Ingredients

- 4 tablespoons farm butter, divided
- 1 large spaghetti squash, deseeded and cut in half lengthwise
- Seasoning to taste
- 2 crushed cloves garlic
- 1 cup onion, sliced up very finely
- 1/2 teaspoon dried Italian seasoning
- 3 ounces wafer-thin salami
- 1/2 cup tomatoes, cut up very finely
- 1/2 cup Kalamata olives, cut in half
- Half a cup of parsley, sliced up very finely
- 4 large eggs

Method

Set your oven to 400. Lay the squash out onto a baking tin/ oven dish, face side up. Spread the face with half the butter and season as you like. Bake until it is tender and cooked through – about three quarters of an hour.

What that is cooking, set your stove to Med-Low. Place the rest of the butter in a heavy-bottomed skillet and let it melt. Add in the garlic, onions and seasoning and fry until the onions start to caramelize. Put the salami and tomatoes in and fry for ten minutes or so, stirring every now and again.

Add the olives and remove from the heat. Scrape out the squash's flesh and mix with the tomato mixture. Make four deep depressions in the tomato mixture and crack an egg into each one. Put into the oven and cook until the eggs are done to your liking.

9. Special Breakfast Omelet

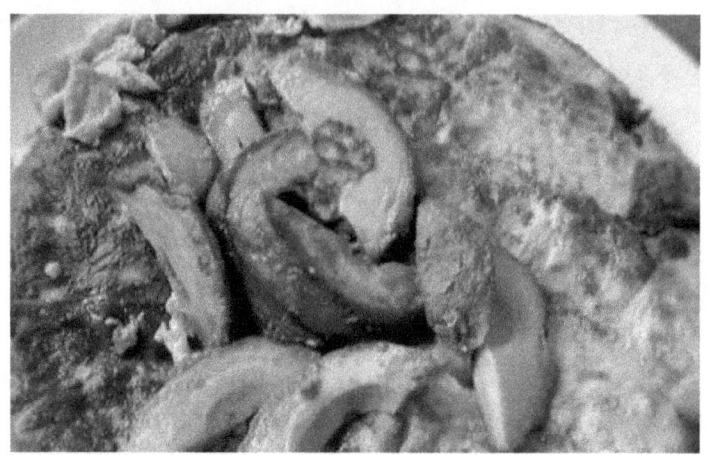

Serves 4

Ingredients

- 10 Kalamata olives, stones removed
- 4 eggs
- 2 Ounces of Brie
- 2 tablespoons MCT Oil
- 1 teaspoon mixed herbs
- 2 tablespoons farm butter
- 1 avocado
- ½ teaspoon table salt

Method

Using a big bowl, mix the MCT oil, eggs, herbs, salt and olives well. Peel the avocado and slice up thickly. Set your stove to

High and place the butter in a non-stick skillet to melt. Fry up the avocado slices until they are a little golden all over.

Take out of the pan and put to one side. Put the eggs into the same pan and thinly slice the Brie so that it is evenly distributed. It won't stay on the top. Put a lid on and continue to fry for two or three minutes or till golden underneath. Flip it over and cook for another couple of minutes. Serve with the avocado on top.

10. Coconut Porridge

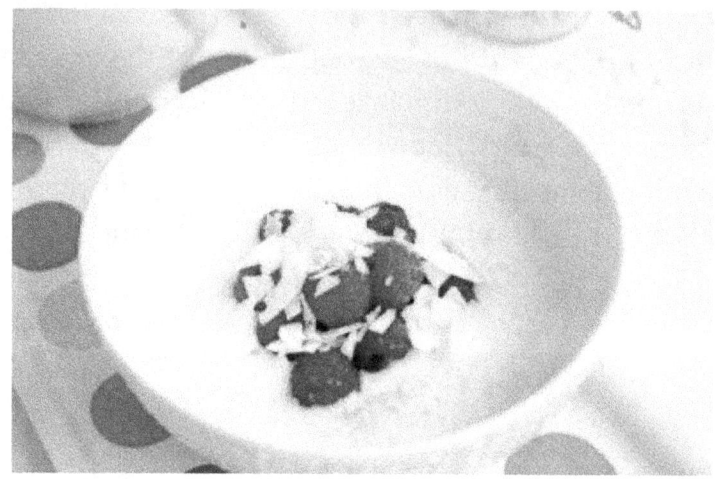

Serves 1

Ingredients

- 1 egg
- 7/8 ounces of farm butter
- 1 tablespoon coconut flour
- 1 pinch salt
- 4 tablespoons coconut cream
- 1 pinch psyllium husk powder

Method

Set your stove to Low and mix up everything well. Put into a heavy-bottomed saucepan and cook until it reaches the thickness that you want. Stir it all the time. You can serve with the milk of your choice and fresh fruit.

11. Egg and Asparagus Breakfast

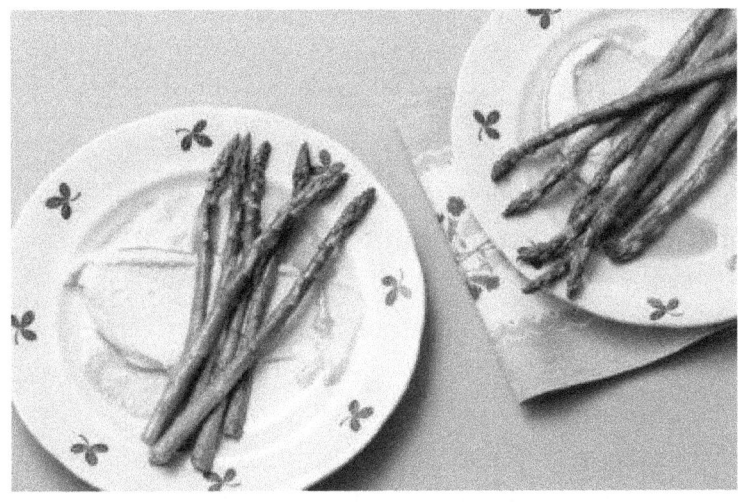

Serves 2

Ingredients for Eggs

- 4 eggs
- 2 ounces of farm butter
- 3¼ ounces of fresh parmesan, grated
- Seasoning to taste
- 8 tablespoons sour cream

Ingredients for Asparagus

- 1 tablespoon olive oil
- 3¼ ounces of farm butter
- 1½ pounds fresh asparagus
- 1½ tablespoons lemon juice

Method

Set your stove to Medium and let the farm butter melt in a frying pan. Scramble the eggs in the same pan. As soon as done, blend the eggs with the sour cream and the cheese until you have a creamy sauce. Season as you like. Set your heat to Medium. In a clean pan – a griddle pan works particularly well, heat up the olive oil. Cook the asparagus until just done. Season as you like.

Set your stove to Medium and add the farm butter. Heat until it starts to go brown and starts to smell a little nutty. Take it off the stove and allow to cool slightly before adding your lemon juice. Put back on the heat at Medium and put the asparagus in with the butter and heat until heated throughout. Plate and serve with the eggs on top.

12. Tuna and Caper Salad

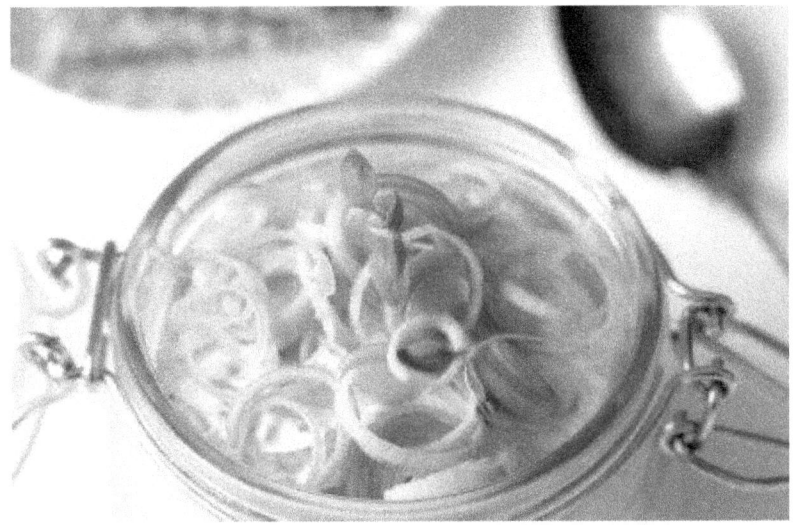

Serves 2

Ingredients

- 8 tablespoons mayo
- 1 can tuna packed in olive oil
- 2 tablespoons sour cream
- 3 – 5 leeks, chopped up nice and fine
- Seasoning to taste
- 1 tablespoon capers
- Chili flakes if you want them

Method

Drain the tuna and mix in the rest of the ingredients and you are done.

13. Caprese Omelets

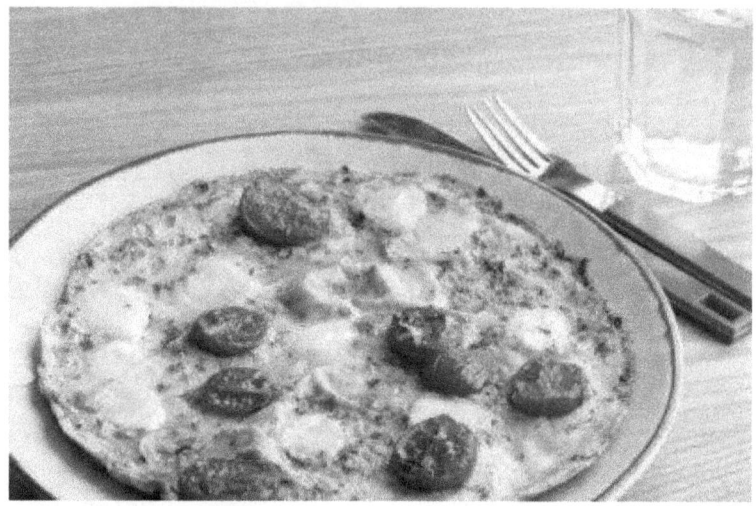

Serves 2

Ingredients

- 6 eggs
- 2 tablespoons olive oil
- 3½ ounces of cherry or Roma tomatoes, halved
- ⅓ pound fresh mozzarella
- 1 tablespoon chopped up nice and finely fresh basil or half the amount of dried basil
- Seasoning to taste

Method

Mix together the eggs and seasoning well and then stir in the basil. Halve the tomatoes and slice up the cheese. Set your stove to Med-High and warm the oil in a big frying pan. Add the tomatoes and fry until they start to soften. Add in the egg and, when that has firmed slightly before putting the cheese on top. Set the heat down to Med-Low and cook until done.

14. Spinach Frittata

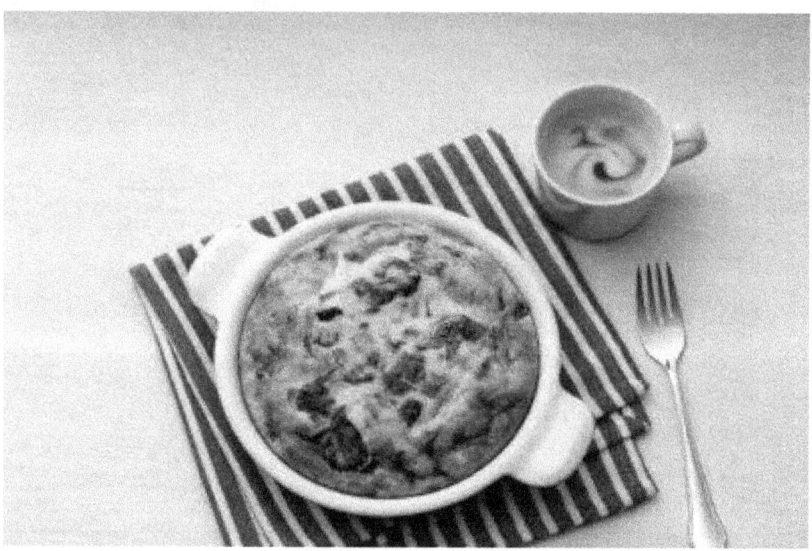

Serves 4

Ingredients

- 1 cup double cream
- 8 eggs
- ½ pound fresh spinach, chopped up nice and finely
- 1/3 pound cheese, grated
- 1/3 pound chorizo or bacon, diced
- 2 tablespoons farm butter
- Seasoning to taste

Method

Set your oven to 350. Set your stove to Med-High and melt the butter in a pan. Add the bacon and fry until nice and crispy. Put the spinach in and allow to wilt a little. Fry the bacon in farm butter until crispy. Add the spinach.

In a bowl, mix the cream and eggs well. Grease an oven-proof dish and put the egg mixture into it. Mix in the rest of the ingredients and bake for about half an hour.

15. Egg Spread

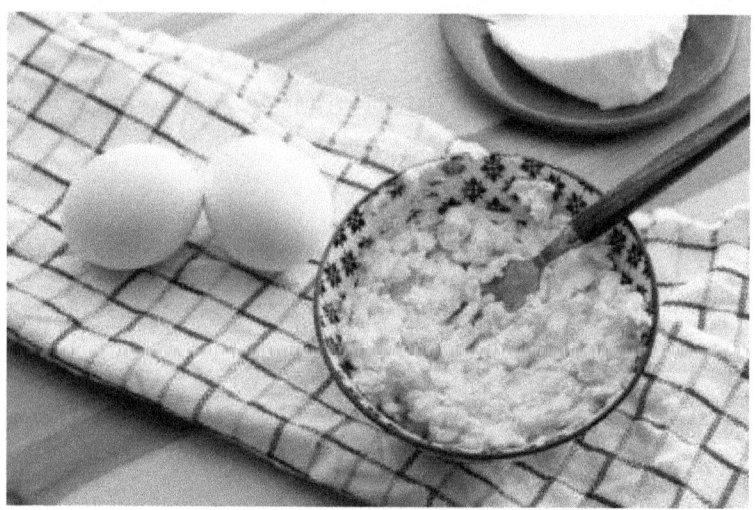

Serves 2

Ingredients

- ⅓ pound farm butter
- 4 eggs
- Seasoning as required

Method

Set your stove to Medium. Fill a pot with enough water to cover all of the eggs. Boil until the eggs are hard boiled (around eight minutes once the water has started to boil.) Plunge into cool water and peel once cool to the touch. Slice the eggs up finely and cream with the farm butter and seasoning. This makes a good topping for low-carb bread.

I hope that you are enjoying this book so far, and if you could spare 30 seconds, I would greatly appreciate you leaving a review on Amazon.com.

Chapter 2

Lunch

1. Lemon Butter Salmon

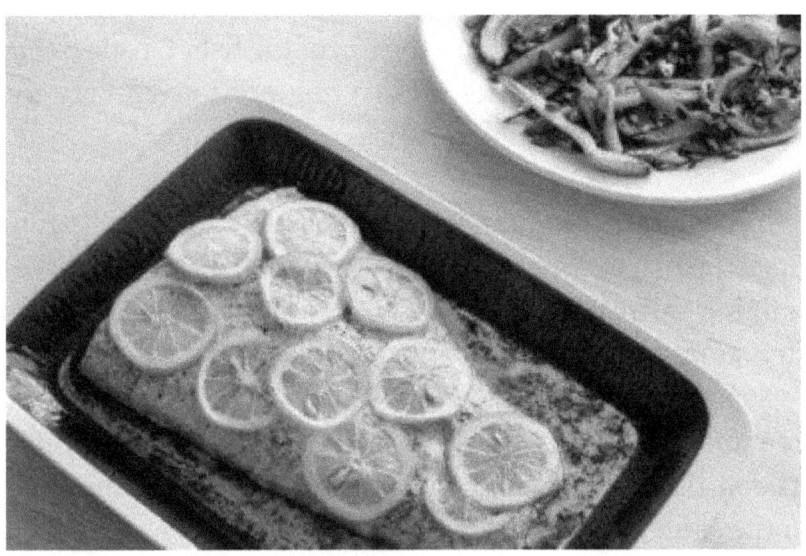

Serves 6-8

Ingredients

- 2¼ – 3 pounds salmon
- 1 tablespoon olive oil
- 1 lemon
- 1 teaspoon table salt
- 7 ounces of farm butter
- Powdered black pepper

Method

Set your oven at 400. Grease and oven-proof dish with olive oil and put the salmon into it with the skin side facing the base of the dish. Add seasoning as you like. Slice up the lemon as thinly as possible.

Place the lemon slices all over the top of the fish. Divide the farm butter in two equal portions. Slice one portion up very thinly and place on top of the lemon slices.

Place on your oven's middle rack and cook for about 25 minutes or until the fish is done. Set the stove to Med-High and place the remaining farm butter into a smaller pot and cook until the butter starts to froth.

Take it off the stove and allow it to cool a little. Add lemon juice a little at time until well incorporated. Serve the lemon butter with the salmon and whatever side dish you like.

2. Thai Fish with Curry and Coconut

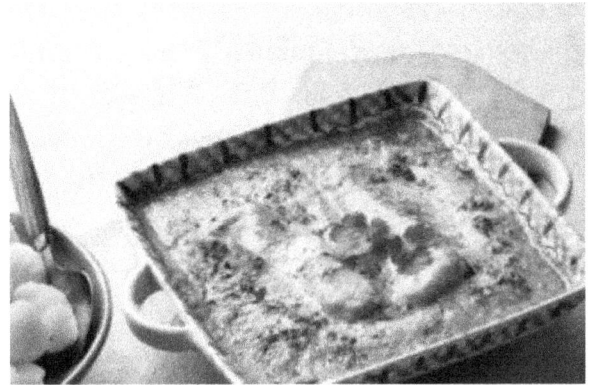

Serves 4

Ingredients

- Seasoning to taste
- 1½ pounds white fish or salmon
- 4 tablespoons farm butter
- 1 can coconut cream
- 1 – 2 tablespoons red curry paste or green curry paste
- 8 tablespoons freshly picked cilantro, chopped
- 1 pound broccoli
- farm butter to grease the oven-proof dish

Method

Set your oven at 400. Grease an oven-proof dish with some butter. Use a dish that the fish just fits into – you do want the fish to fill the width and length of the dish. Place the fish in the oven-dish and season to taste. Divide the farm butter up evenly over the fish.

Mix together the curry paste, cilantro and coconut cream well and then pour it over the fish. Put in the oven and cook for around 20 minutes or so. The fish must be cooked throughout. Boil up the broccoli in the interim. Cook on the stove in water that has been salted lightly until just done. Serve along with the fish.

3. Salmon with Pesto and Spinach

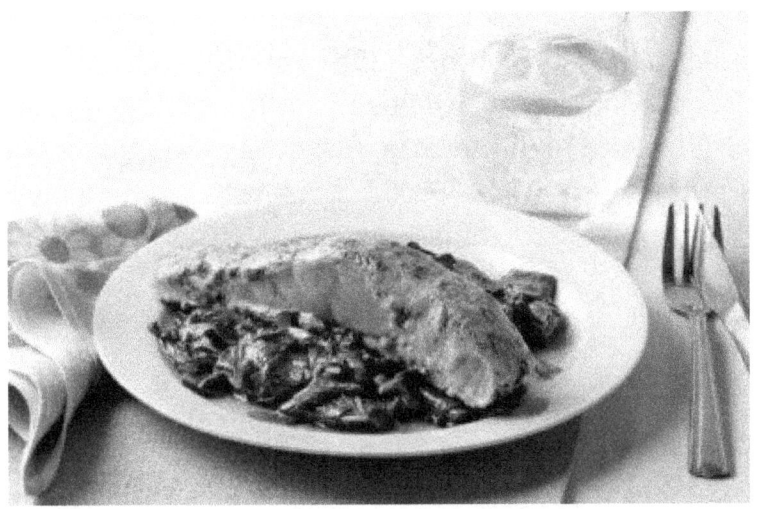

Serves 3

Ingredients

- 1 cup mayo or sour cream
- 1½ pounds salmon
- 1 tablespoon green pesto
- 1 pound fresh spinach
- Seasoning to taste
- 2 ounces of fresh Parmesan, grated
- 1 ounces of farm butter

Method

Set your oven at 400. Grease an oven-proof dish and place the salmon in it, with the skin side facing the base of the dish.

Season to taste. Mix together the pesto, Parmesan and the mayo well and then spread evenly over the salmon pieces.

Put in the oven and cook for about 15 minutes or till the salmon is cooked through. While the fish is in the oven, set your stove to Med-High and melt the farm butter. Fry the spinach, coating in the butter until it just wilted. Season as you like and serve with the fish on the top of it.

4. Mushroom and Fish Oven Bake

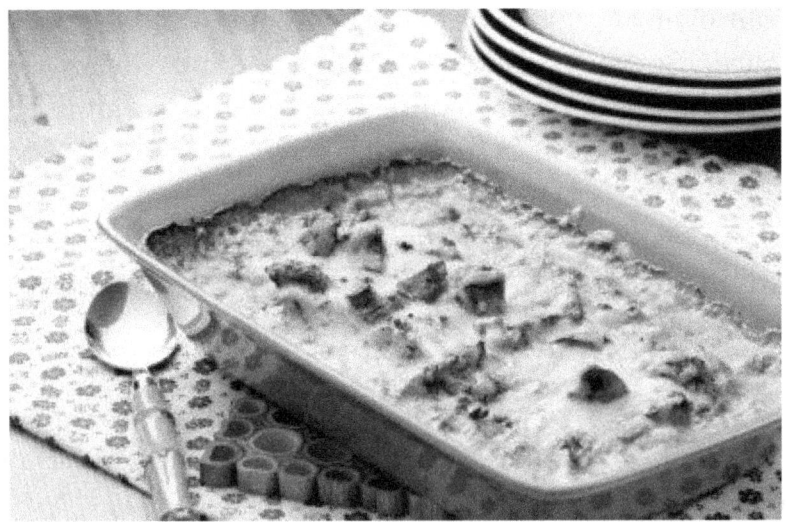

Serves 4

Ingredients

- 3¼ ounces of farm butter
- 1 pound mushrooms
- 1 teaspoon table salt
- 2 tablespoons freshly picked parsley, coarsely picked
- Pepper, to taste
- 2 cups double cream
- ½ pound cheese, grated
- 2 – 3 tablespoons Dijon mustard
- 1½ pounds white fish, for example cod
- 3¼ ounces of farm butter

Method

Set your oven at 350. Clean the mushrooms and then cut them into slices. Set your stove to Med-High and put the farm butter in a heavy-based frying pan until it melts. Add your mushrooms and cook until they have softened.

Season to taste and add in the parsley. Add the double cream and stir in the mustard. Reduce the heat to Low and cook slowly until the sauce is thickened and reduced.

Grease an oven-proof dish. Season the fish as you like and place it in the dish. Take about ¾ of the cheese and top the fish with it. Pour the mushrooms on top.

Finish off with the remaining cheese and then put into the oven. Put in the oven for about twenty minutes to half an hour or until the fish is just done throughout. Serve with cauliflower "rice".

5. Foil-Baked Fish

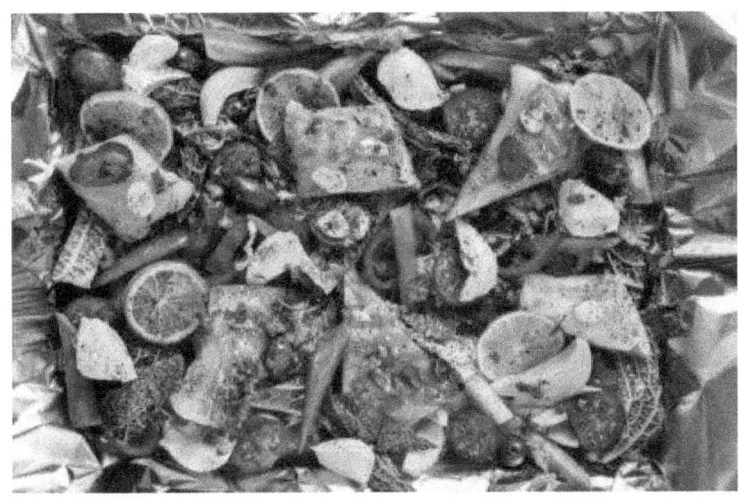

Serves 4

Ingredients

- ½ leek
- 2 pounds white fish filets
- 1 mild onion
- 2 red bell peppers
- 2 – 3 garlic cloves
- 12 cherry tomatoes
- 1 carrot
- 1 fresh bulb of fennel
- 6¾ tablespoons olives, pitted
- 1 lime, sliced
- Fresh thyme or freshly picked parsley
- ⅓ pound farm butter
- Seasoning to taste

- 2 – 3 tablespoons olive oil
- 6¾ tablespoons white wine

Ingredients for Quick Aioli

- Seasoning to taste
- 1 garlic clove, crushed
- 1 cup mayo

Method

Set the oven at 400. Take a roasting dish and place foil into it. You want enough foil so that you are able to make a tent over the fish and veggies. Chop up the fish and put it into the center of the foil. Slice up the veggies and put them in the foil as well. Season to taste and add the spices.

Drizzle wine and then oil over the top. Put some of the farm butter on top of that. Close off the tent of foil – seal tightly. Put in the oven and cook for about 35 minutes. Make the aioli by mixing together the garlic and the mayo. Add seasoning to taste. Serve with the fish and veggies.

6. Buttery Fish and Veggies

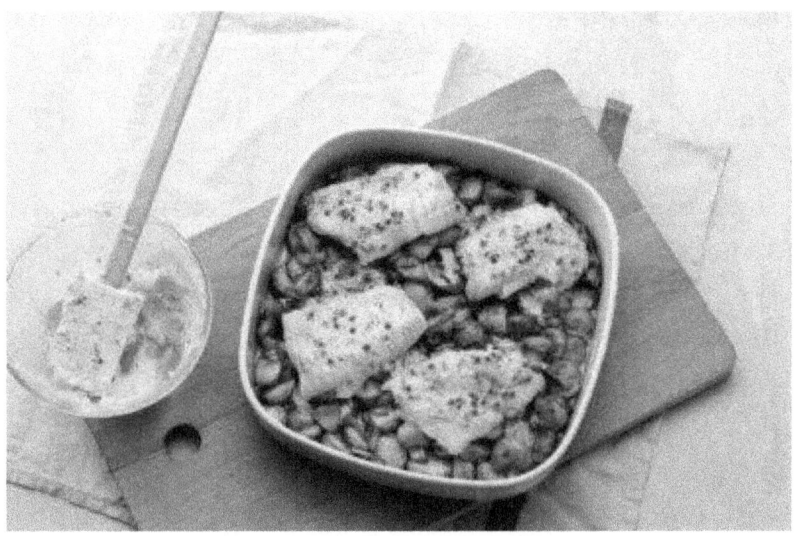

Serves 4

Ingredients

- 1 pound of Brussel Sprouts
- 1½ pounds cod or hake
- 7 ounces of mushrooms
- ½ teaspoon dried thyme
- 2 – 3 tablespoons small capers
- 1 tablespoon olive oil
- Seasoning to taste
- 1 ounce of farm butter, to fry the fish in Pink Herbed Farm Butter
- ½ garlic clove
- 1⁄3 pound farm butter, at room temperature
- ½ teaspoon lime juice

- ¼ teaspoon table salt
- 2 ounces of fresh Parmesan, grated
- 1 tablespoon pink pepper

Method

Start by making the butter. Crush the pepper up coarsely and blend into the butter, along with the lime juice. Set your oven at 400. Grease an oven-proof dish. Halve the Brussels sprouts and put them into the dish in a single layer. Drizzle the olive oil over them and season as required. Put them in the oven for about 15 minutes.

Halve the mushrooms. Set your stove to Med-High and melt the farm butter. Add the mushrooms and the thyme and fry until the mushrooms start to soften. Put the capers in and cook for a little while longer. Season as you like.

Take the Brussels sprouts out of the oven and put the mushrooms over the top. Adjust the seasoning as required and put the fish onto the veggies. Top with lots of the farm butter mixture. Put into the oven and cook for around 20-25 minutes or so.

7. Thai Cabbage and Salmon

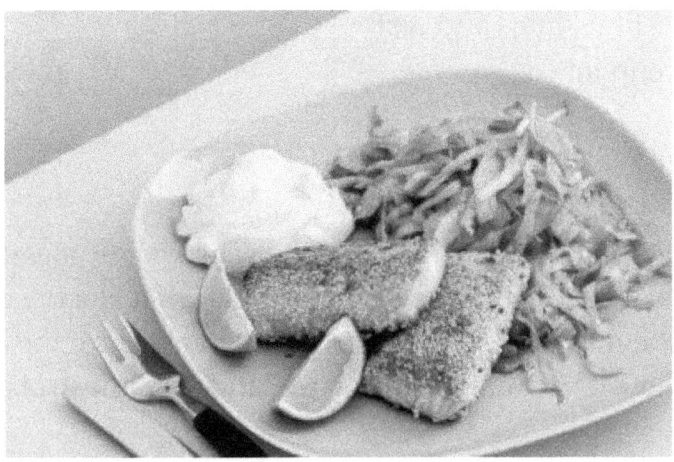

Serves 4

Ingredients for the Salmon

- 2 tablespoons Sesame seeds
- 1½ pounds salmon pieces
- 3¼ ounces of farm butter
- 1 lime to serve with the fish
- Seasoning to taste

Ingredients for the Cabbage

- 2 pounds cabbage, grated
- 2 tablespoons coconut oil
- 1 tablespoon red curry paste
- Seasoning to taste
- 1 tablespoon sesame oil

Ingredients for the Lime mayo

- ½ lime, juice and zest
- 1 cup mayo

Method

Make the lime mayo first. Add the ingredients together and season to taste. Place in the fridge while you make the cook the rest of the meal. Set your stove to High and place the coconut oil into a wok. Stir in the curry paste and then the cabbage.

Fry quickly till the cabbage starts to brown but still has a bit of crunch. Season as you like. When the cabbage is almost done, you should add the oil and stir it well. Put aside in the warmer drawer.

Season the salmon as you like and then dip it into the seeds so that they are completely coated. Set your stove to Med-High and melt the farm butter in a heavy-based frying pan. Fry up the salmon for a few minutes, flip and cook on the other side.

Reserve the left-over butter to serve over the meal. Plate the cabbage and serve with the salmon. Drizzle the butter over the salmon and serve the lime mayo on the side and a portion of fresh lime.

8. Fish and Low-Carb Chips

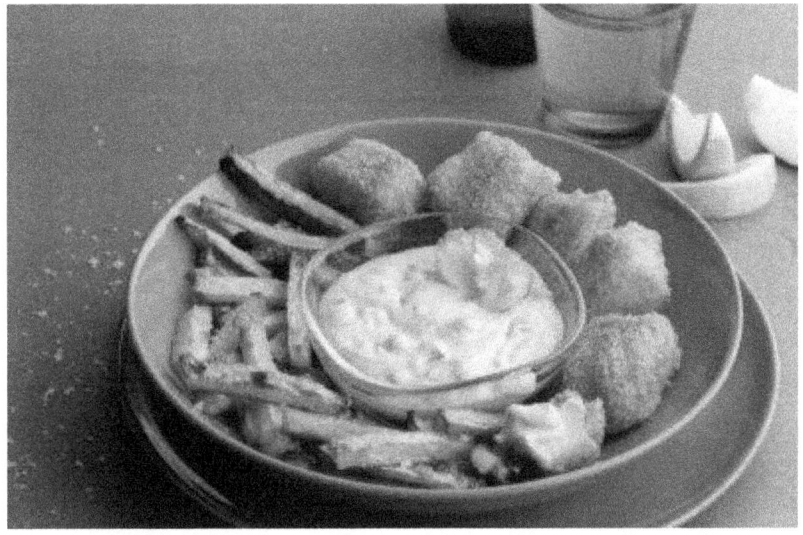

Serves 4

Ingredients

- 1½ pounds white fish
- 1½ pounds rutabaga, peeled
- 2 eggs
- 1 cup fresh Parmesan, grated
- 1 cup almond flour
- 1 teaspoon paprika
- 1 teaspoon table salt
- ½ teaspoon onion powder
- ¼ teaspoon pepper
- 1 lemon, for serving
- 2 cups oil to fry the food in

Ingredients for the Tartar sauce

- ½ tablespoon curry powder
- ¼ cup dill pickle relish
- 1 cup mayo

Method

Start by making the tartar sauce. Store in the refrigerator when cooking the rest of the food. Set your oven at 400. Line a baking tin with baking paper. Slice the rutabaga into very thin julienne strips. Brush them with the oil and place onto the baking sheet. Season as you like and place in the oven. Cook for about half an hour or until done. In the interim, get the fish ready. Beat the eggs until frothy.

On a separate plate, mix together the cheese and flour and season as you like. Cube the fish into one inch pieces and dip into the flour mixture. Dip it into the eggs and then recoat in the flour mixture. When the oil is hot, deep fry the fish for about five minutes or so or till the coating is a nice brown color. Serve along with the chips and the sauce.

9. Tropical Salmon and Cabbage

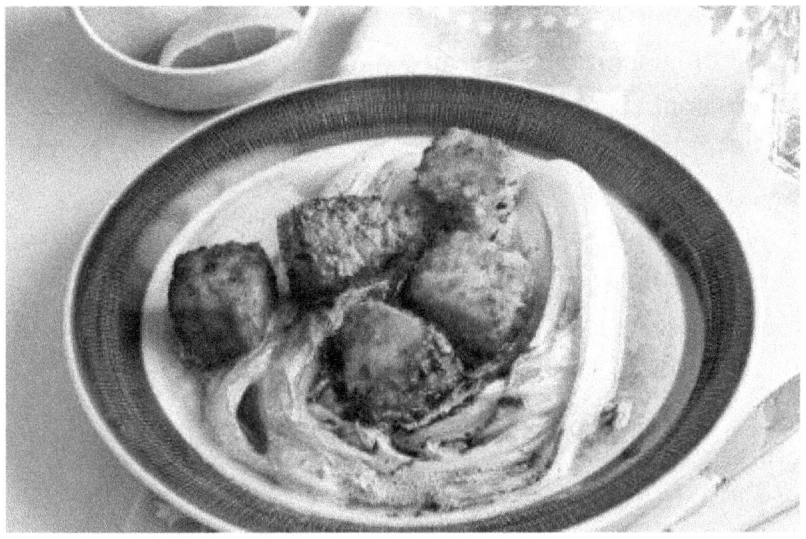

Serves 4

Ingredients

- 1 tablespoon olive oil
- 1 1/3 pounds salmon
- 1/2 cup desiccated coconut
- 1 teaspoon table salt
- 1 teaspoon turmeric
- 3 1/3 tablespoons olive oil, to fry in
- 1/2 teaspoon onion powder
- 1 1/3 pounds cabbage
- Lemon, to serve with
- Seasoning to taste
- 4 ounces of farm butter

Method

Cube the salmon into one-inch cubes. Drizzle with the oil. Mix together the coconut, onion powder, salt and turmeric on a side plate and coat the cubes of salmon. Set your stove to Med-High and fry the cubes till they are a nice golden color. Set aside in your warmer drawer.

Chop the cabbage up into wedges. Set your stove to Med-High and melt the farm butter in a heavy-based frying pan. Add the cabbage, season to taste and fry until cooked and it starts to caramelize. Serve up the cabbage and salmon and use any remaining butter as a sauce for the cabbage. Add a lemon wedge for each plate and you are done.

10. Prosciutto and Salmon

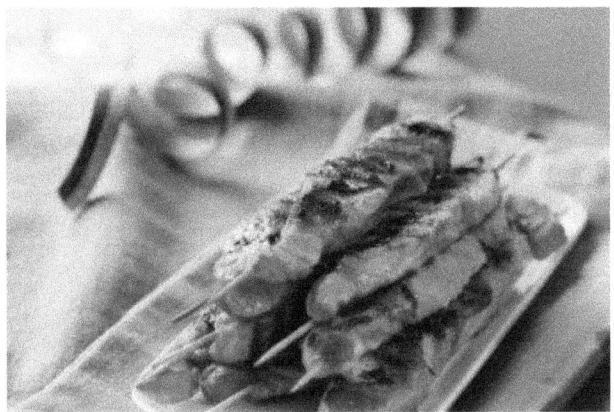

Serves 4

Ingredients

- 1 1/3 pounds salmon
- Freshly picked basil, chopped up nice and finely
- 1 pinch powdered black pepper
- 1 tablespoon olive oil
- 8 wooden skewers
- 3¼ ounces of prosciutto, in slices

Method

Put the skewers into cool water and allow them to become fully saturated. Cube the salmon into one-inch cubes and thread onto the skewers. Roll each skewer in the pepper and basil mix. Chop up the prosciutto into long strips and wrap it around the fish. Brush with the oil and cook under a hot grill or in a hot frying pan.

11. Fish Soup with Saffron

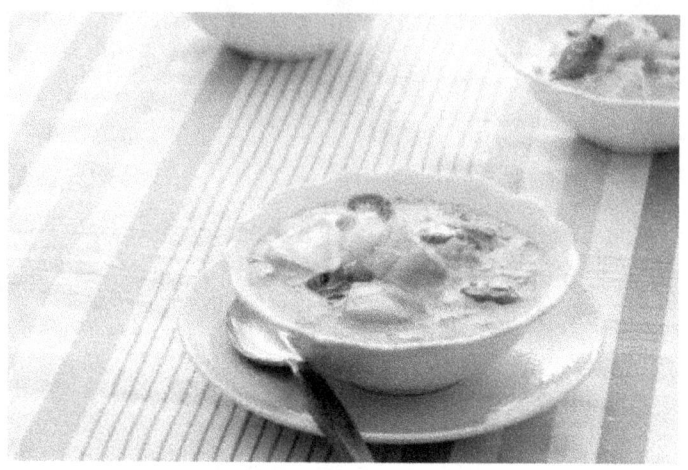

Serves 4

Ingredients

- 2 garlic cloves, chopped up nice and finely
- 1 mild onion, chopped up nice and finely
- 1 bulb of fresh fennel, chopped up nice and finely
- 1 pinch saffron
- ½ tablespoon tomato paste
- 2 cups water
- 1¼ cups sour cream
- 2 fish or veggie bouillon cubes
- The juice of 1 lime
- 8 cherry tomatoes
- Seasoning to taste
- Freshly picked parsley, chopped up nice and finely
- 1½ pounds one- inch pieces of white fish

Ingredients for the Aioli

- 1 tablespoon freshly picked parsley, chopped
- 1 – 2 garlic cloves, crushed
- ½ cup mayo

Method

Set your stove to Medium and fry the onion, fennel, saffron and garlic until the onions start to turn translucent. Use a pot that will be able to contain all the ingredients. Stir in the tomato paste. Halve the tomatoes and add them as well. Fry for a couple of minutes.

Mix the bouillon cubes to a little boiling water so that they dissolve. Stir in with the rest of the water and add to the pot. Let the mixture come to a boil and then reduce the heat to Low. Let it simmer for 5-10 minutes until the liquid reduces. Season as you like.

Mix the lime juice in and then add the sour cream and let the soup come to a boil again. Stir in the fish and allow it to simmer for another 5 or 10 minutes or until the fish is completely done. While the fish is cooking, make the Aioli. Mix up the mayo, parsley and the garlic and serve alongside the soup.

12. Salmon Cured in Apples

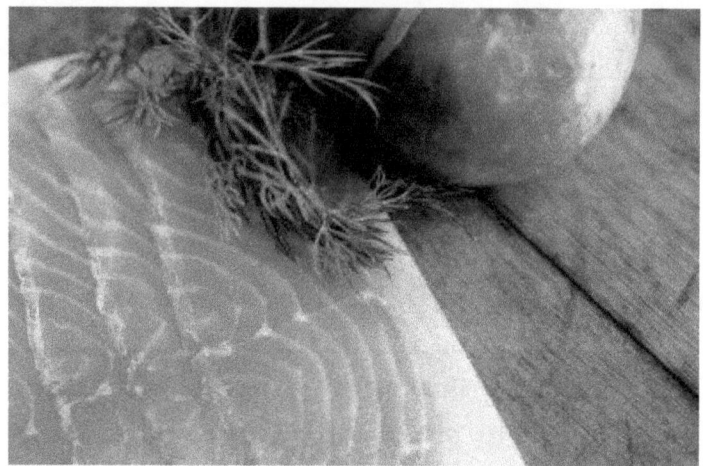

Serves 4

Ingredients

- 3 tablespoons salt
- 1 pound salmon, taken from the mid-section of the fish
- 2 – 3 tablespoons calvados (you can leave these out if you prefer)
- 1 tablespoon peppercorns, crushed a little
- A bunch of fresh dill
- 2 apples

Method

Make sure that the salmon is properly deboned. Grate up the apples and coarsely chop the dill. Mix together the dill and the apples and layer half of the mixture in a deep dish that the salmon will fit into. Take the salt and pepper and mix together.

Rub about half of this into the salmon skin. Put the salmon on the apple mixture, skin side down. Rub what is left of the salt mixture into the salmon and cover it with what is left of the apple mixture.

If you want to intensify the taste of the apples, add the Calvados. Wrap the salmon in cling wrap and put something heavy on top of it – such as a jar of jam. Place on a plate in the refrigerator for two days.

After this time, you can remove the salmon and discard the apple mixture. Slice up the salmon thinly and serve with mayo that has been mixed with a little finely chopped dill and some mustard.

13. Yellow Beets with Anchovy Salad

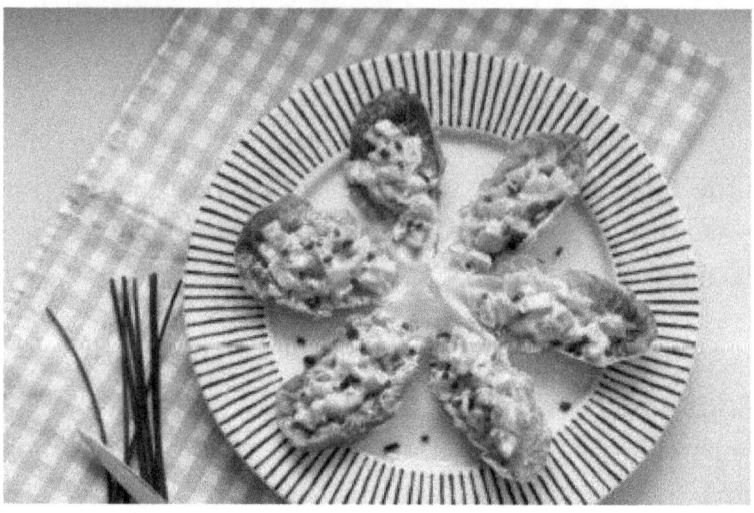

Serves 2-4

Ingredients

- 2 ounces of anchovies
- ½ pound yellow beets, cooked
- ½ red onion
- 2 endives
- 1 cup mayo
- Fresh chives

Method

Chop up the beets finely. Do the same for the onions and anchovies. Mix with the mayo and the chives and serve on the lettuce leaves.

14. Fish and Beetroot Bake

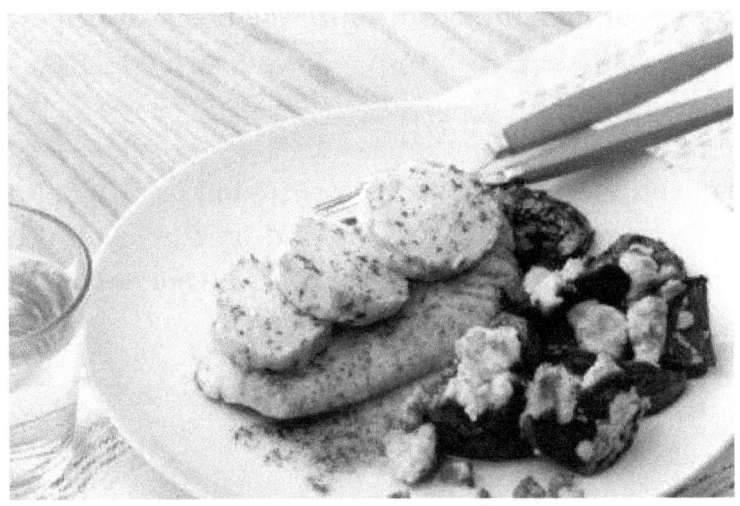

Serves 4

Ingredients

- 2 – 3 tablespoons farm butter to fry the fish in
- 1¾ pounds white fish
- 1 pound beetroots
- 3 tablespoons olive oil
- 1⁄3 pound feta or blue cheese
- 1⁄3 pound herbed farm butter
- Seasoning to taste

Method

Set your oven at 400. Clean the beetroots well, peel them and then quarter them. Grease an oven-proof dish and place the beetroots in a single layer. Season as required, bearing in mind that the cheese is also quite salty. Crumble the cheese over the top and finish off by drizzling the oil over the top. Put in the oven for about half an hour or until the beetroots are done. If the cheese is getting too brown, you can turn down the heat a little at about 10 minutes to go.

In the meantime, you can set your stove to Med-High. Melt the farm butter in a heavy-based pan and fry the fish until done. Season to taste. Serve with the beetroot and herbed farm butter on the side.

15. Chicken Tonnato

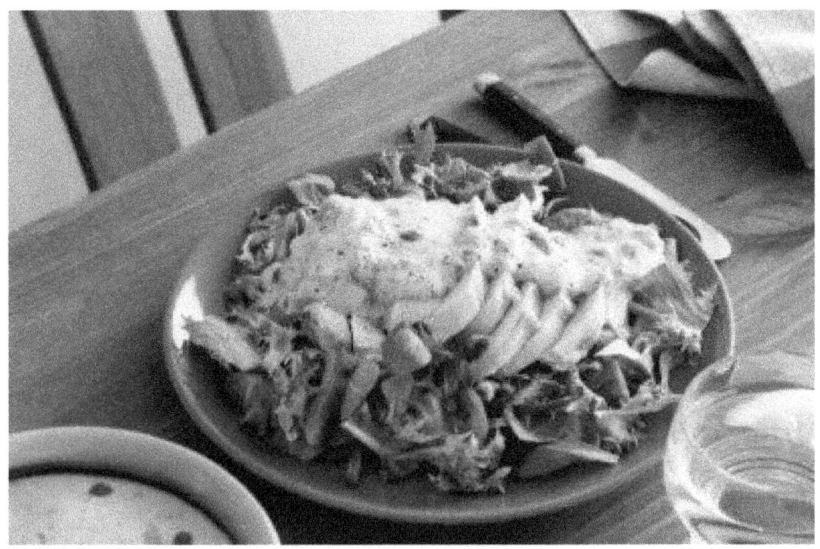

Serves 2

Ingredients for the Tonnato sauce

- 1 can tuna packed in olive oil
- 2 tablespoons small capers
- 2 garlic cloves
- 1 teaspoon dried parsley
- ¼ cup freshly picked basil, chopped up nice and finely
- 2 tablespoons lemon juice
- ¼ cup olive oil
- ½ cup mayo
- ¼ teaspoon powdered black pepper
- ½ teaspoon table salt

Ingredients for the Chicken

- water
- 7 ounces of leafy greens
- 1½ pounds chicken breasts
- salt

Method

Start off with the sauce. Mix together all the sauce ingredients and blend until smooth. Set aside. Now make the chicken. Set your stove to Med-High. Put the chicken into a pot and cover with enough water to submerge it completely. Season to taste. Let the water come to a boil and then reduce the heat to Medium and let it cook for 15 minutes or so till the chicken has cooked through.

As an alternative, you can use cooked chicken leftover from a roast and skip this altogether. The chicken should be left to rest for around 15 minutes before you slice it into bite-sized pieces. Serve on top of some leafy greens and with the sauce over the top of the chicken. Serve with some fresh, quartered lemon.

Once again, thank you for reading this book, and I hope you're getting a lot of valuable information. I would greatly appreciate it if you could take 30 seconds to leave me a review for this book on Amazon.com.

16. Avocado, Bacon and Goat-Cheese Salad

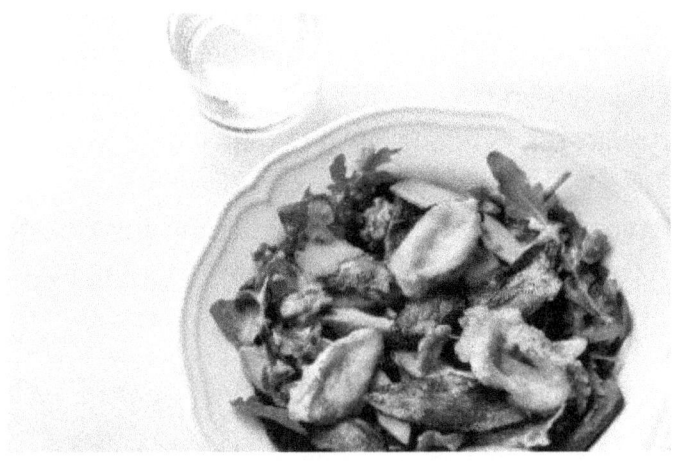

Serves 2

Ingredients

- ½ pound bacon
- ½ pound mild goat cheese
- 2 avocados
- 4 ounces of lettuce
- 4 ounces of walnuts

Ingredients for the Dressing

- 2 tablespoons double cream
- ½ cup mayo
- The juice of ½ lemon
- ½ cup olive oil

Method

Set your oven at 400. Line a baking sheet with baking paper. Cube up the goat cheese and then place on the baking sheet. Place on the uppermost rack in the oven until it turns a nice golden color. Set your stove to Med-High and fry up the bacon in a heavy-based frying pan until it is nice and crispy.

Cube the avocado and top the lettuce with it. Put the cheese and bacon on top. Top off with the nuts. Mix together all the ingredients for the dressing and season to taste. Blend well and serve with the salad.

17. Coleslaw

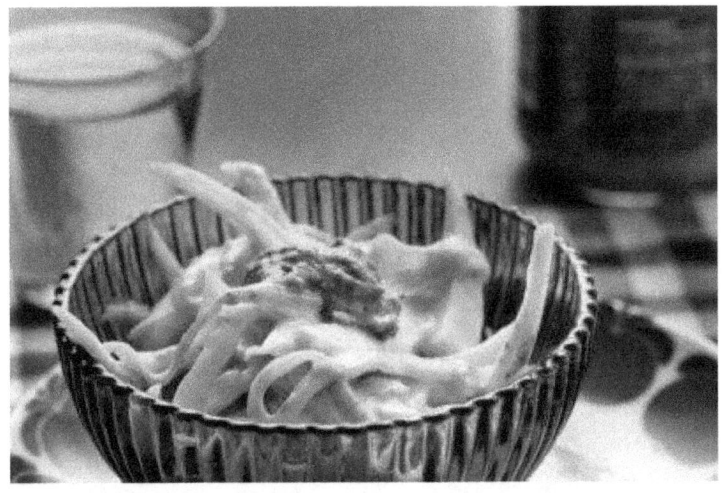

Serves 1

Ingredients

- The juice of ½ lemon
- ¼ green cabbage, coarsely grated
- 1 teaspoon table salt
- 1 pinch fennel seeds
- 6¾ tablespoons mayo
- 1 tablespoon Dijon mustard
- 1 pinch pepper

Method

Mix together the cabbage, lemon juice and the salt. Put aside for about 10-15 minutes. Drain off any liquid and then mix in the remaining ingredients.

18. Fennel and Lemony Pea Roast

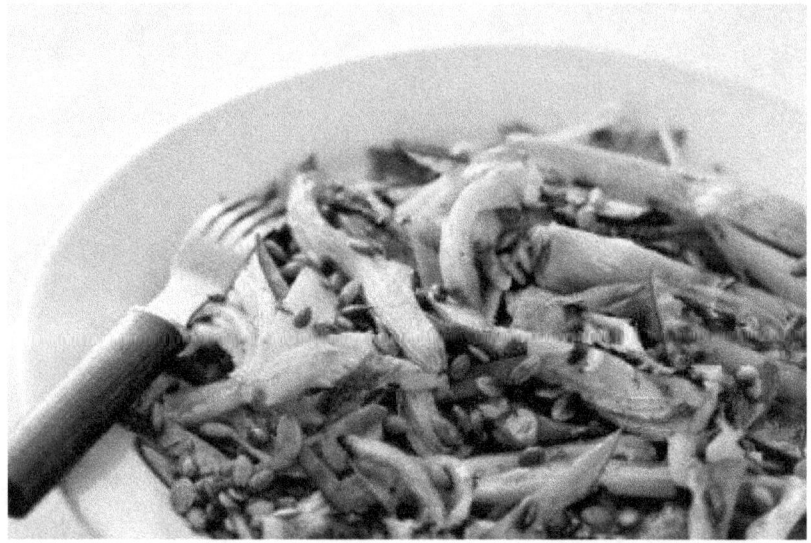

Serves 4

Ingredients

- 4 fresh fennel bulbs
- 1 lemon
- 3 tablespoons olive oil
- 2 tablespoons pumpkin seeds, roasted
- 1/3 pound sugar snaps
- Seasoning to taste

Method

Set your oven at 450. Slice up the fennel into wedges and layer in an oven-proof dish. Drizzle with the oil and season as you like. Squeeze the juice out of the lemon and then cut the rest of the lemon into wedges. Place it in amongst the fennel. The wedges are there mainly to flavor the dish, you can discard them after cooking if you don't want to eat them. Place in the oven for about half an hour or until the fennel is soft and starting to caramelize. When the fennel is done, slice the peas and mix with the pumpkin seeds as well.

19. Brussels Sprouts With A Tang

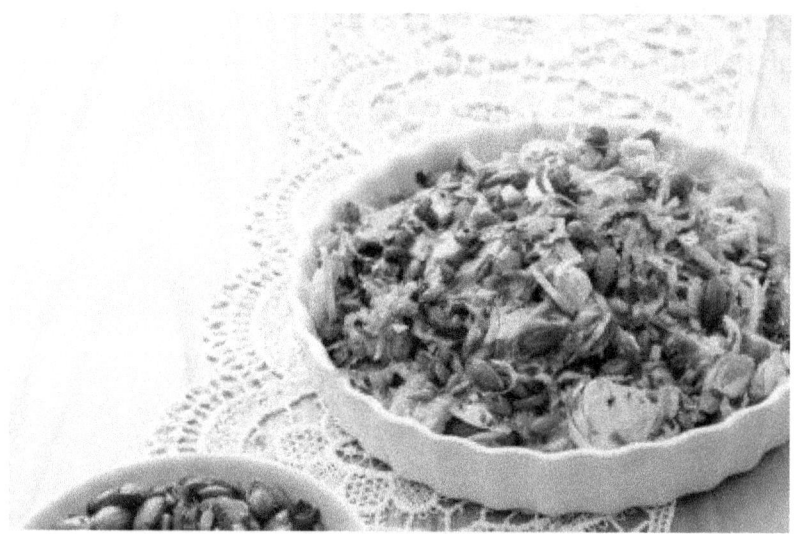

Serves 4

Ingredients

- 8 tablespoons olive oil
- 1 pound Brussel Sprouts
- The zest and juice of 1 lemon
- Seasoning to taste
- ¾ cup of the Seed and Almond mix below

Ingredients for Spicy Seed and Almond Mix

- ½ pound almonds
- 2 tablespoons coconut oil
- 8 tablespoons pumpkin seeds
- 1 tablespoon powdered cumin

- 8 tablespoons sunflower seeds
- ½ teaspoon table salt
- 1 tablespoon chili paste

Method

Clean the Brussels sprouts and slice them up. Put them in a bowl. Mix together the lemon zest, lemon juice and the olive oil. Season to taste and mix with the Brussel Sprouts. Set aside for about ten minutes.

In the meantime, make the Spicy Seed and Almond Mix. Set the heat to Med-High and heat up the oil in a heavy-based frying pan. Stir in the chili and then add the nuts and seeds. Stir well and season to taste. Fry for no more than a minute or two. Serve with the Brussel Sprout salad and store the remainder in a sealed container.

20. Cabbage and Orange Salad

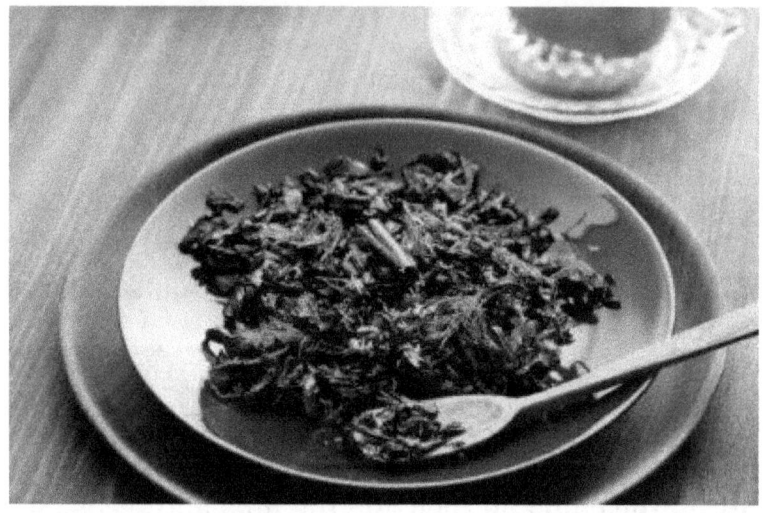

Serves 4

Ingredients

- 4¼ ounces of farm butter
- 2 pounds red cabbage
- 1 teaspoon table salt
- 1 powdered cinnamon stick
- 1 orange, juice and zest
- ¼ teaspoon powdered black pepper
- 1 tablespoon red wine vinegar
- 2 tablespoons fresh dill, chopped

Method

Finely grate the cabbage. Set the stove to Med-High and melt the butter in a heavy-based frying pan. Stir in the cabbage and fry for about 15 minutes or until it has started to go soft and becomes glossy.

Season as you like and mix in all of the other ingredients except for the dill and the orange zest. Reduce the heat to Low and allow the mixture to simmer for about 10 minutes. Stir in the dill and zest just before you serve the cabbage.

21. Eggplant Salad

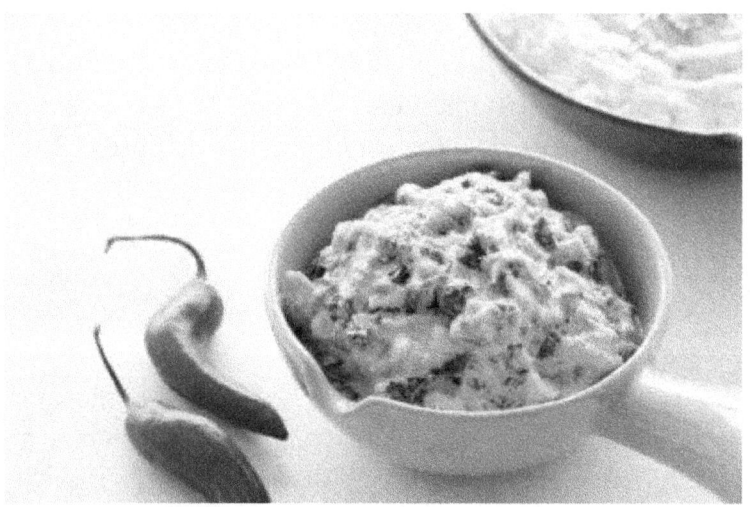

Serves 4

Ingredients

- 2 bell peppers
- 2 eggplants
- 1 red chili pepper
- The juice of 1 lemon
- 1 teaspoon table salt
- 2 garlic cloves
- 6¾ tablespoons mayo

Method

Set your oven at 480°F. Cut the bell peppers and eggplants into two equal halve lengthwise. Remove the seeds from the pepper. Grease an oven-proof dish and lay the peppers and eggplants halves into the dish with the cut side facing down. Place in the center of your oven and cook for 20 minutes. Turn the eggplants over and put everything back in the oven for another 10 minutes. Remove the dish and let the veggies cool for a bit.

Halve the chili and remove the seeds. Cut up the chili extremely finely. Crush the garlic and chop up the fresh parsley. Mix it all together with lemon juice. Skin the veggies from the oven and cube them. Mix the parsley mixture and add the mayo. Place covered in the refrigerator for at least 3 hours, preferably overnight, so that the flavors develop completely.

Enjoying this book?

Check out my other best sellers!

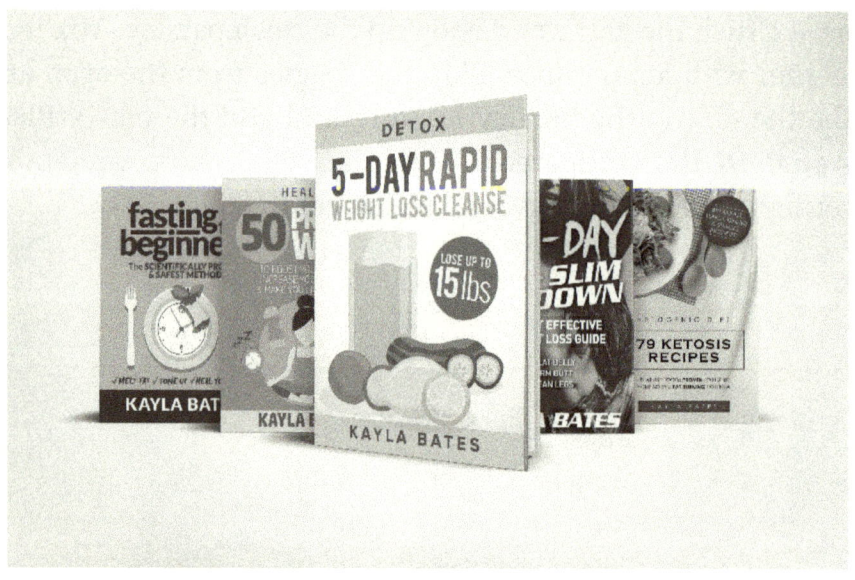

Get your next book on sale here:

TopFitnessAdvice.com/go/Kayla

Chapter 3

Dinner

1. Chicken Stir-Fry

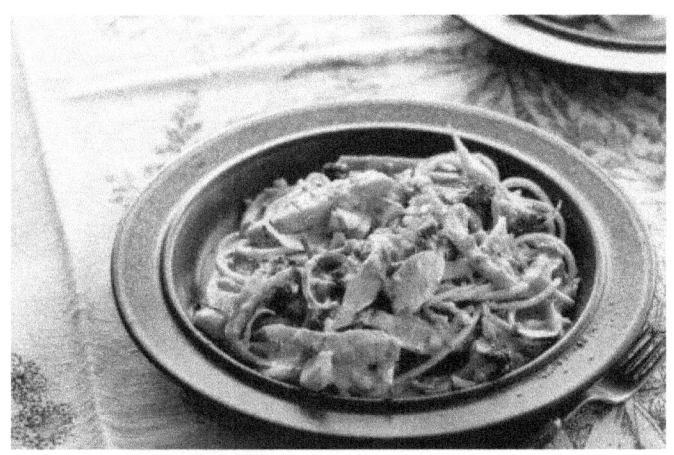

Serves 4

Ingredients

- 5⅓ tablespoons salted peanuts
- 1 pound broccoli
- 2 tablespoons coconut oil
- 1 mild onion
- 1⅔ cups coconut milk
- 1 pound cooked chicken breasts
- 1 – 2 tablespoons green curry paste
- Seasoning to taste
- 1 – 2 tablespoons peanut butter

Method

Chop the onion up into nice, thin rings. Chop up the broccoli, leaving the stems intact as far as possible. Set your stove to High. Heat up the oil in a big wok. Add the onion and cook until it starts to turn translucent. Add the broccoli and cook until just done but with a bit of crunch.

Chop up the chicken and stir in with the broccoli. Set the peanuts aside as a garnish and add all the other ingredients to the pan. Stir well. Cook for a few minutes, stirring often, so that the sauce thickens up. Season as required and serve with the peanuts on top.

2. Brussels Sprouts And Onions

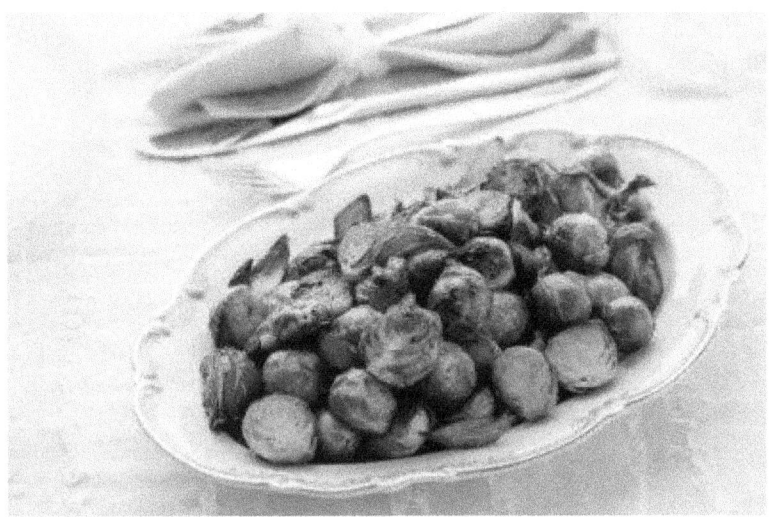

Serves 4

Ingredients

- 1 pound Brussels sprouts
- 2 mild onions
- 4¼ ounces of farm butter
- 1 tablespoon red wine vinegar

Method

Set your stove to Medium and melt the farm butter. Chop the onions into quarters and stir-fry them until they start to caramelize. Stir in the vinegar and the seasoning that you require. Reduce the heat and simmer until the onion is completely soft. Set aside.

Chop the sprouts into halves. Add them to the same pan you fried the onions in, adding more farm butter if necessary. Fry until they are just cooked. Season to taste and mix with the onions.

3. Charcuterie Buffet Platter

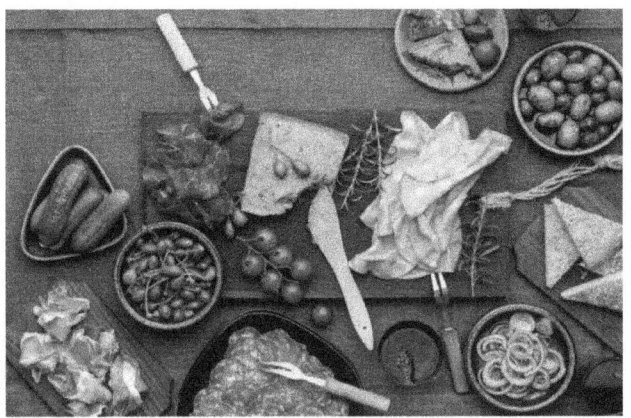

Serves 10

Ingredients

- 4¼ ounces of prosciutto
- 4¼ ounces of salami
- 4¼ ounces of bresaola
- 4¼ ounces of pâté
- 4¼ ounces of mortadella
- 4¼ ounces of olives
- 12 cherry tomatoes
- 4¼ ounces of capers

Method

You can choose whatever cold meats you like but do look for those that are cured without sugar and flavor enhancers. Lay out the meat on a large platter and put the veggies alongside it. Serve with low-carb bread or crackers.

4. Thanksgiving Turkey with Citrusy Butter

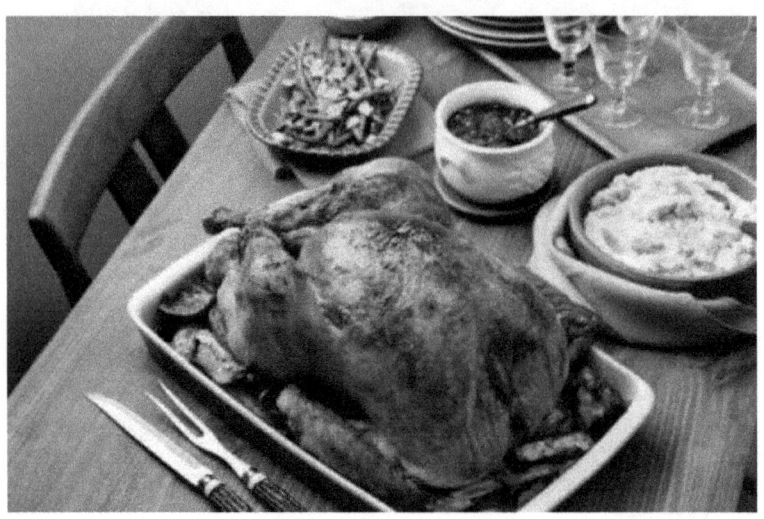

Servings 12

Ingredients for the Turkey

- ⅔ pound root celery, peeled and chopped up
- 13 pound whole turkey
- 2 carrots, peeled and chopped
- The turkey giblets
- 2 mild onions, chopped up
- 2 tablespoons olive oil
- 1 teaspoon powdered black pepper
- 1 cup of plain water
- The juice of 1 orange
- 2 teaspoons salt

Ingredients for the Citrusy Farm Butter

- 2 shallots, chopped up nice and finely
- ⅔ pound farm butter, softened
- ¼ teaspoon powdered black pepper
- 2 sprigs of freshly picked sage, chopped up nice and finely
- 1 teaspoon table salt
- The zest of 1 orange

Stuffing

- 2 mild onions, chopped up nice and finely
- 2 tablespoons farm butter
- ½ pound root celery, diced
- ⅓ pound bacon, diced
- 1 apple, grated
- 2 pieces of low-carb bread
- 2 ounces of pecan nuts, chopped
- 2 pounds ground pork
- 1 cup double cream
- ½ teaspoon ground nutmeg
- 1 tablespoon farm butter, to grease the oven-proof dish
- 2 sprigs of freshly picked sage, chopped up nice & finely
- ½ teaspoon powdered black pepper
- 1 teaspoon table salt

Ingredients for the Gravy

- 3¼ ounces of cream cheese
- 1 – 2 cups double cream

- 1 – 2 cups turkey pan juices

Method

Start by making the citrusy butter. Blend all the ingredients for the butter together until well-combined. Slip two thirds of the butter under the skin of the turkey thighs and breasts. Move on to the stuffing. Set your stove to Med-High and melt the butter in a large frying pan. Fry the onion until it starts to soften.

Add in the bacon and the root celery. Cook until the root celery becomes golden. Take off the heat and add the apple and the pecans. Leave so that it can cool. Mix together the beef and spices with the onion mixture.

Grease an oven-proof dish and put two-thirds of the stuffing mixture into it. The rest will be used to stuff the turkey. Cook the stuffing for about half an hour or until the meat is done. Set your oven at 350. Season the turkey as you like. Stuff the turkey and then tie the thighs together. Grease a large roasting pan and place the turkey into it, with the breast facing up.

Put the giblets and the other veggies around the turkey. Season as you like. Drizzle the veggies with olive oil and put the sage on top. Add a cup of water as well. Put the remaining citrusy farm butter on top of your turkey. Add the orange juice as well.

Cover the turkey breast and wings with foil to prevent them from drying out too much. Place the turkey into your oven and cook for between 4 and 5 hours – the cooking time will depend on how big your chicken is.

Do check on the turkey once an hour or so basting it when you do. You may need to add more water. When there is just an hour to go, take off the foil. Take out of the oven and veggies and place in a foil tent so that it can rest for at least 20 minutes before being carved.

Use the juices from the roasting pan to make the gravy. You will need about two to three cups of liquid so if there is not enough, you need to add water. Set your stove to High and bring the pan juices to a boil. Reduce the heat to Low and stir in the cream and cream cheese. Simmer until the gravy is nice and thick.

5. Slow Cooked Roasted Pork and Gravy

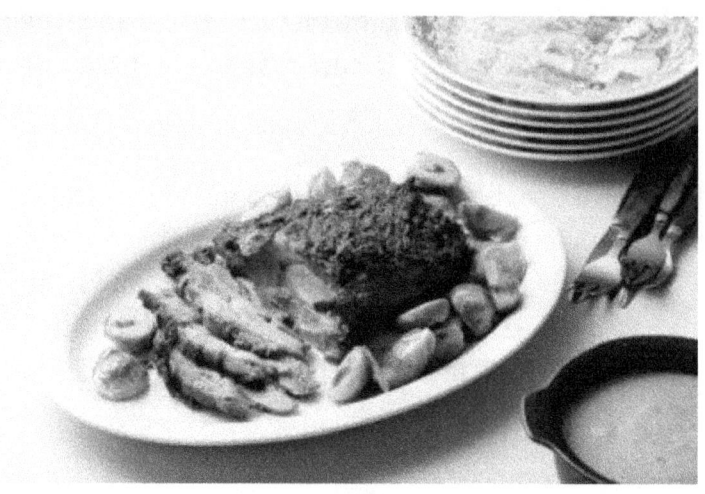

Serves 6

Ingredients

- ½ tablespoon salt
- 2 pounds pork roast
- 1 bay leaf
- 2½ cups water
- 5 peppercorns
- 2 teaspoons dried thyme
- 1 ⅓ ounces of fresh ginger
- 1 tablespoon paprika powder
- 2 garlic cloves
- 1 tablespoon olive oil
- ½ teaspoon powdered black pepper

Creamy Gravy

- 1½ cups double cream
- Juices from the roast

Method

Set your oven at 200. Grease an oven-proof dish. Season the meat as required and put enough water in so that 2/3 of the roast is covered. Add the pepper and the bay leaf. Cook for between 7 and 8 hours, or until cooked throughout.

Set the stove to 450. Remove the remaining juices from the dish and keep for the gravy. Mix together the finely chopped ginger and the garlic. Stir in the pepper, herbs and oil. Brush the roast with the mixture and put it back in the oven for about 15 minutes.

Gravy: Put the juices through a sieve and discard the solids. You will need three cups of pan juices – if you don't have enough, add water. Put into a saucepan. Set your stove to Medium and bring the juices to a boil until the liquid is reduced by half. Stir in the cream. Allow it to come to a boil and then reduce the heat to Low. Allow it to cook gently until it is as thick as you like it, stirring often.

6. Green Beans Side Dish

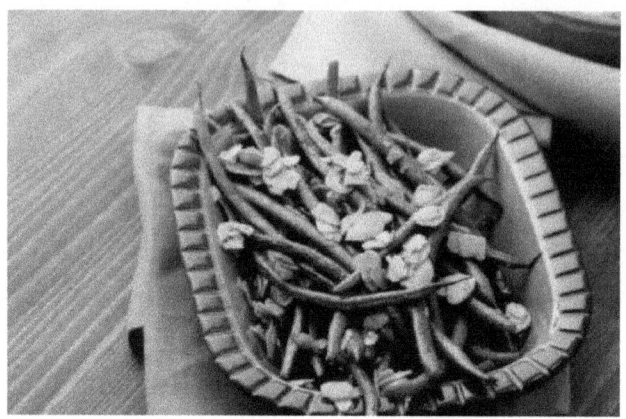

Serves 6

Ingredients

- 3 tablespoons farm butter
- 4 garlic cloves, crushed
- 3 tablespoons olive oil
- ½ teaspoon table salt
- 5 ⅓ tablespoons almonds, slivered
- 1½ pounds fresh green beans
- ¼ teaspoon powdered black pepper

Method

Clean the beans and trim them. Set the stove to High and melt the farm butter along with the oil in a heavy-based frying pan. Add in the garlic and cook for a minute. Set your stove to Med-High and put the beans in. Cook until done – about 5 minutes. Stir in the almonds. Season to taste.

7. Bacon Farm Butter

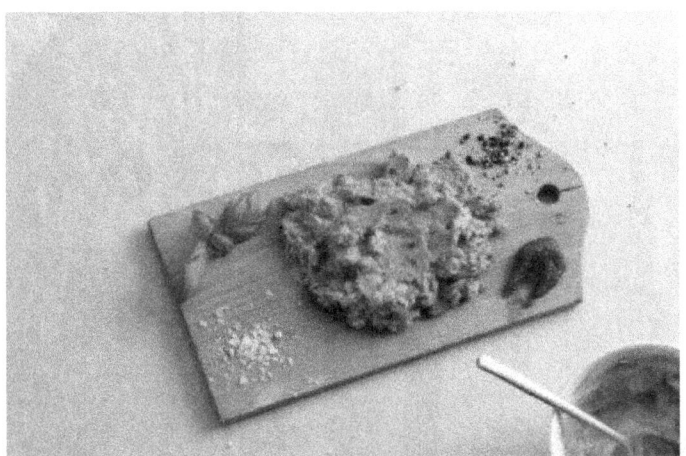

Serves 4

Ingredients

- 2 shallots
- 4¼ ounces of farm butter
- 2 ounces of bacon
- 1 teaspoon tomato paste
- 1 tablespoon fresh basil

Method

Chop the shallots up nice and finely. Chop the bacon into little bits. Set the stove to Med-High and melt a tablespoonful of the farm butter. Cook the bacon and the shallots and cook until the bacon is crisp and the shallots are cooked. Set aside to cool. Mix together the tomato paste, the basil and the farm butter. Wrap the butter in baking paper so and role it into shape.

8. Colorful Roast Veggies

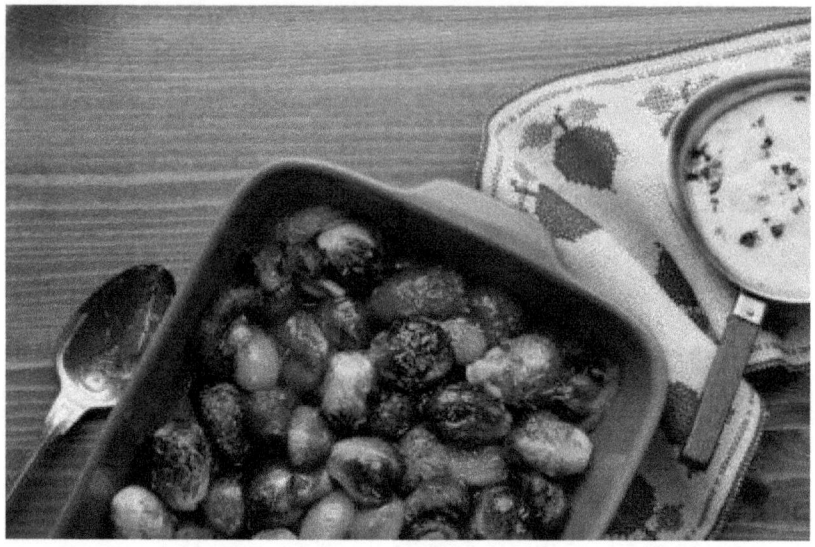

Serves 6

Ingredients

- 8 tablespoons olive oil
- ½ pound cherry tomatoes
- 1 pound Brussels sprouts
- ½ pound mushrooms
- ½ teaspoon powdered black pepper
- 1 teaspoon table salt
- 1 teaspoon dried thyme

Method

Set your oven at 400. Clean the veggies and chop them up so that they are equally sized. Grease an oven-proof dish and put the veggies into it in a single layer. Pour the olive oil over the top and put the spices on as well.

Put in the oven and cook for about half an hour or until the veggies are cooked throughout.

9. Chicken with Satay Sauce

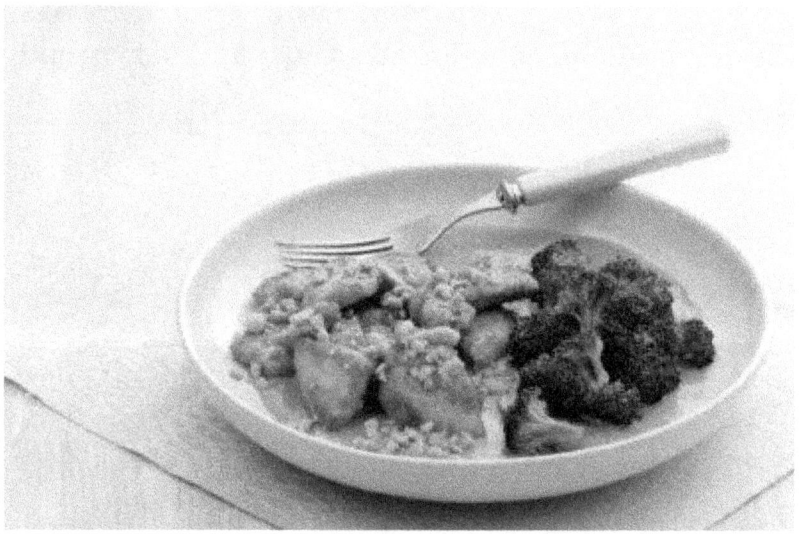

Serves 4

Ingredients

- ½ teaspoon table salt
- 1 tablespoon fresh ginger, crushed
- 1½ pounds chicken thighs
- 1 teaspoon turmeric
- 3 tablespoons coconut oil
- 1 tablespoon coriander seeds

Ingredients for Satay sauce

- 1 – 2 red chili peppers, deseeded and chopped up nice and finely
- 1⅔ cups coconut cream

- 1 garlic clove, chopped up nice and finely
- 6 – 8 tablespoons peanut butter
- 3⅓ tablespoons soy sauce

Method

Put the oil, coriander, turmeric and ginger into a sealable bag. Chop the chicken into 1-inch pieces and put them into the bag as well. Shake until the chicken is properly coated and set aside to marinade for at least 15 minutes.

While waiting for that, you can make up the satay sauce. Set your stove to Med-High. Put all of the ingredients for the sauce into a little pot and allow it to come to a boil.

Reduce the heat and cook until the sauce is nice and thick. Season as required. Set the stove to High. Heat up some oil in a wok and brown the chicken. Add seasoning to taste and reduce the heat. Cook the chicken until it is done throughout. Serve the chicken with the sauce and garnished with peanuts.

10. Sweet Potato Fries

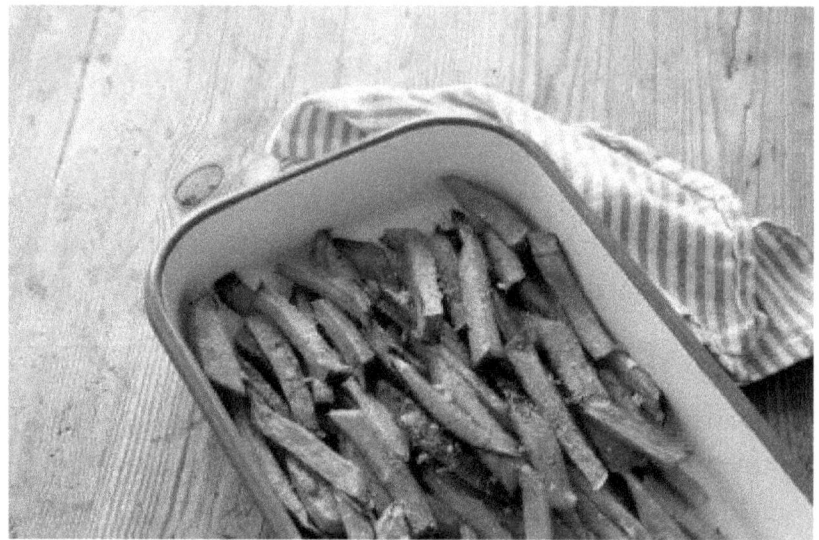

Serves 4

Ingredients

- Seasoning to taste
- 4 tablespoons coconut oil, melted
- 1 pound sweet potatoes

Method

Set your oven at 400. Peel all the potatoes and slice them into fries. Grease an oven-proof dish and layer the fries in one layer. Drizzle the coconut oil over the fries. Stir to coat well. Season to taste and put in the oven for about half an hour or until the fries are cooked through.

11. Sticky Chicken Wings

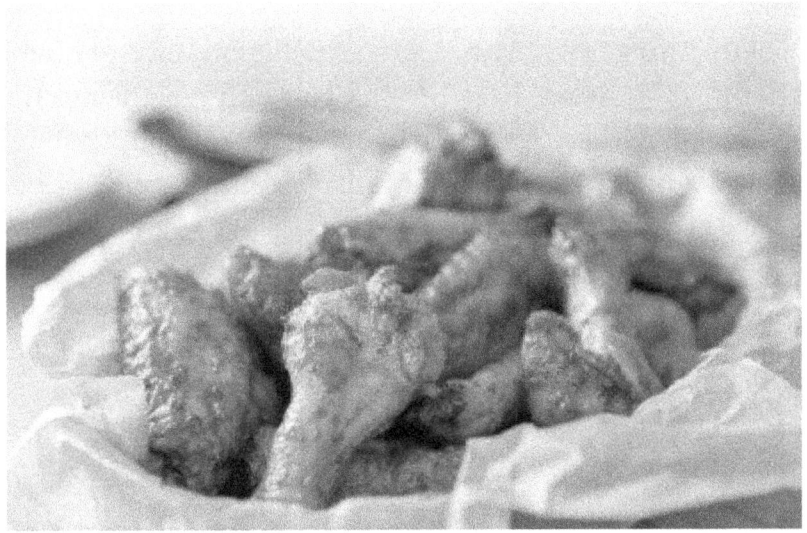

Serves 4

Ingredients

- ¼ teaspoon chili flakes
- 1½ teaspoons table salt
- 2¼ pounds chicken wings
- ¾ cup coconut aminos
- ¼ teaspoon onion powder
- ¼ teaspoon ground ginger
- ¼ teaspoon garlic powder

Method

Set your oven at 450. Grease an oven-proof dish and lay the wings out in a single layer. Season to taste and put into the oven.

Cook for about three quarters of an hour or until cooked through.

In the meantime, work on the sauce. Set your stove to Medium. Warm up a big, heavy-based frying pan and put the aminos in it. Stir in the garlic flakes, ginger, pepper flakes and the onion powder. Bring the sauce to a boil, stirring quite often. Cook until the sauce is thick and sticky. Pour over the wings and make sure that they are coated evenly.

12. Pumpkin Soup

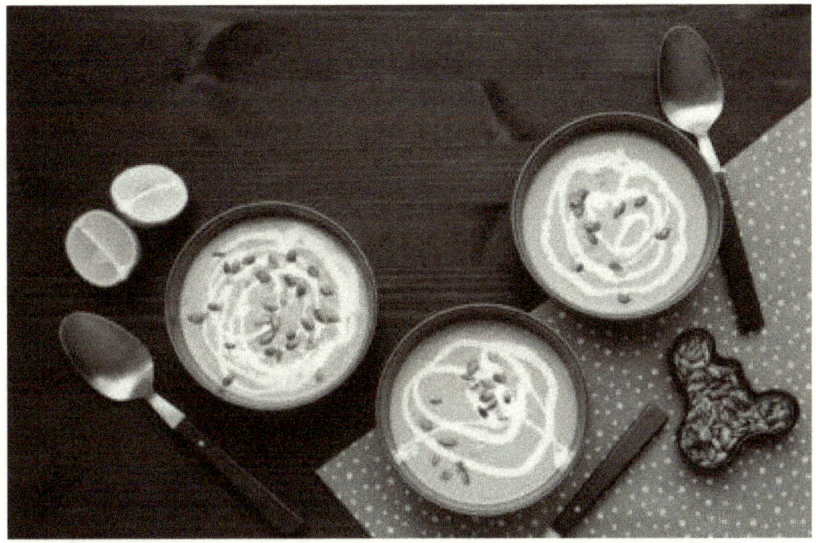

Serves 4

Ingredients

- 2 garlic cloves, crushed
- 2 onions
- ⅔ pound pumpkins
- 2 tablespoons olive oil
- ⅔ pound rutabaga
- 1 teaspoon table salt
- ½ lime, the juice
- 2 cups vegetable stock
- ½ teaspoon powdered black pepper
- ½ pound farm butter

Ingredients for Toppings

- 4 tablespoons roasted pumpkin seeds
- ¾ cup mayo

Method

Set your oven at 400. Peel and cube the pumpkin. Peel and cube the turnip as well. Peel the onion and cut it into thick wedges. Grease an oven-proof dish and lay the veggies in it in a single layer. Season to taste and sprinkle the garlic over the top of it. Drizzle the olive oil over the top.

Put into the oven and cook for about half an hour or until the veggies are cooked through. Set your stove to Med-High. Place the stock and the veggies into a pot. Bring everything to the boil. Reduce the heat to Low and let the soup simmer until it has thickened up.

Stir in the butter and stir until completely incorporated. Take it off the heat and blend the soup until smooth. Stir in the lime juice and herbs. Adjust the seasoning as required. Add a dollop of mayo just before serving and use the pumpkin seeds as croutons.

13. Mashed Broccoli

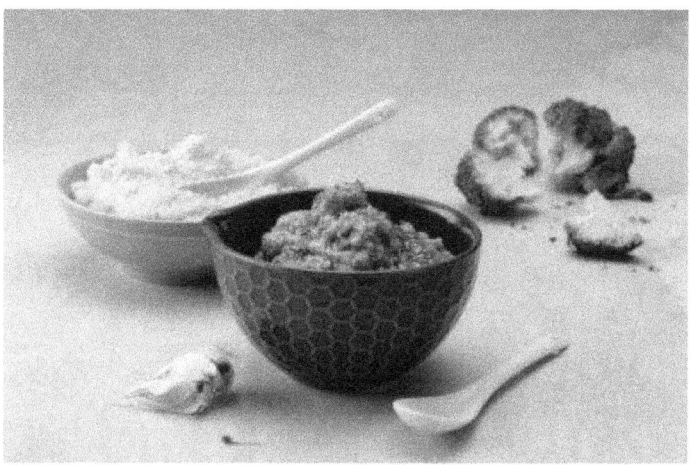

Serves 4

Ingredients

- 4 tablespoons freshly picked parsley, chopped up nice and finely
- 1½ pounds broccoli
- 3½ ounces of farm butter
- Seasoning to taste
- 1 – 2 garlic cloves, crushed

Method

Put the broccoli and garlic into a pot and put enough water in the pot to cover it. Season as required. Set your stove to High and boil the broccoli until it is soft. Drain off as much water as possible and adjust the seasoning if necessary. Add the butter and parsley and blend until it has a smooth consistency.

14. Bone Broth

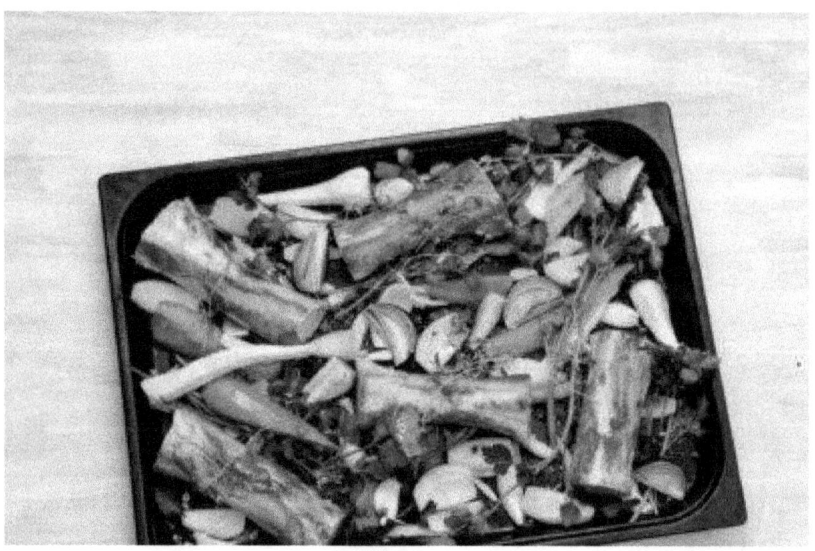

Serves 4

Ingredients

- 2 – 3 onions, peeled and chopped up nice and finely
- 4½ – 6⅔ pounds beef lamb bones
- 2 carrots, peeled
- 2 tablespoons olive oil
- 1 whole head of garlic, peeled and crushed
- 2 tablespoons tomato paste
- 2 tablespoons apple cider vinegar
- Fresh thyme to taste
- Seasoning to taste
- 1 – 2 cups water, have extra on hand to use when boiling veggies

Method

Set your oven at 450. Grease an oven-proof dish and lay the bones and veggies out in a single layer. Add the garlic over the top and season to taste. Mix the olive oil and the tomato paste and cover the bones with the mixture.

Place in the oven with a cup of water. Cook for an hour to an hour and half, topping up the water as necessary. Set your stove to Med-High. Transfer the bones, veggies and any leftover liquid into a pot.

Mix in the vinegar and add enough water to completely submerge everything. Bring to the boil and cook for 15 minutes. Reduce the heat to Low and leave it to simmer for 8 hours. Cook until the broth has a rich flavor and strain. Store what you don't use in the refrigerator or freeze it for use later.

Others who are considering purchasing this book would love to know what you think. If you could spare a few seconds, they would greatly appreciate reading an honest review from you. Simply visit the page on Amazon.com.

15. Hearty Chicken and Butternut Squash

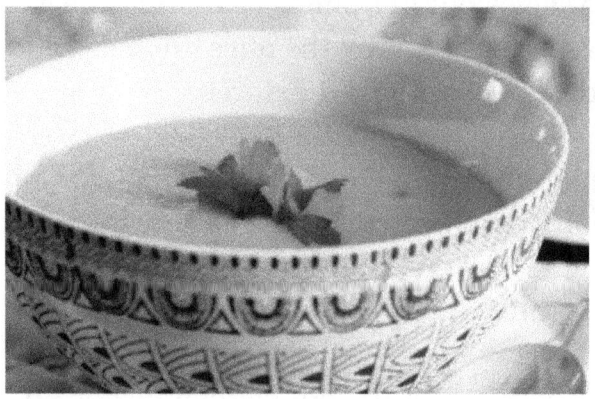

Serves 4

Ingredients

- 6¾ tablespoons coconut oil
- 2 pounds butternut squash
- ½ – 1 teaspoon table salt
- 5 pieces of fresh ginger
- ½ teaspoon chili flakes
- 2 garlic cloves
- 1 tablespoon turmeric
- 1 leek, chopped up nice and finely
- 1⅔ cups chicken, pre-cooked and shredded
- 6¾ tablespoons chicken stock
- 1⅔ cups water
- 2 cups coconut cream
- 1 lime, the juice

Method

Set your oven at 350. Peel the squash and cut into bite-sized pieces. Grease an ovenproof dish and put the squash in it in a single layer. Season to taste and sprinkle with the chili. Put into the oven and cook for about half an hour or until softened.

Peel the garlic and crush it. Peel the ginger and grate it. Set your stove to Med-High and put the coconut oil into a large pot. Fry the garlic, leek and ginger until they soften.

Stir in the turmeric and fry for a couple of minutes. Stir in the squash and the chicken stock. Add the coconut cream. Heat until it comes to a boil and then reduce the heat to Low. Allow the soup to cook gently for half an hour and then blend it until smooth. Add the lime juice and adjust the seasoning if necessary.

Warm the chicken in a little stock either on the stove or in the microwave. Divide it between four bowls and add the soup. Garnish with cilantro and serve.

16. Chicken Coconut Curry

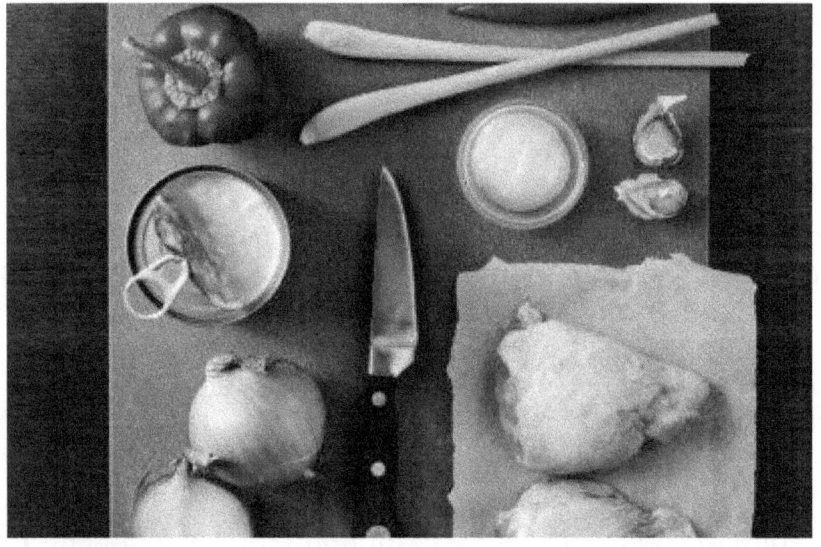

Serves 4

Ingredients

- 2 tablespoons coconut oil
- 2 stalks of lemongrass
- 1 tablespoon curry powder
- 2 mild onions
- 1 can coconut cream
- 1⅓ pounds chicken thighs, boneless
- 1 thumb-sized piece of fresh ginger
- 1 – 2 red bell peppers, sliced
- 2 garlic cloves, crushed
- ½ red chili pepper, chopped up nice and finely

Method

Crush the lemongrass stem. Chop the chicken up into bite-sized pieces. Set your stove to Med-High. Put the coconut oil into a wok and then fry up the curry and the lemongrass. Reduce the heat to Medium and stir in the chicken. Cook until browned all over. Season as required. Remove the chicken from the pan, leave the lemon grass in it.

Chop the onions up nice and finely. Put them into the frying pan and cook until softened. Stir in the coconut cream along with the chicken. Reduce the heat and let it simmer for about 10 minutes or until completely heated through. Take the lemongrass out and throw it out. Serve with the lemon zest.

17. Rutabaga Spirals

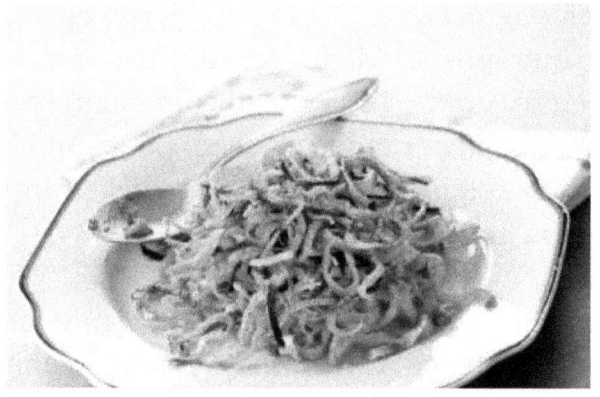

Serves 4

Ingredients

- 5⅓ tablespoons olive oil
- 1½ pounds rutabaga
- 1 teaspoon table salt
- 1 tablespoon paprika

Method

Set your oven at 450. Clean the rutabaga and peel it. Chop into piece that will work with a spiralizer. Alternatively, you can chop them up very finely. Put into a sealable bag. Add the rest of the ingredients and shake well so that the rutabaga is coated. Grease a baking tin and lay out the rutabaga in a single layer. Put it into the oven and cook for about 10 minutes.

18. Huevos Rancheros

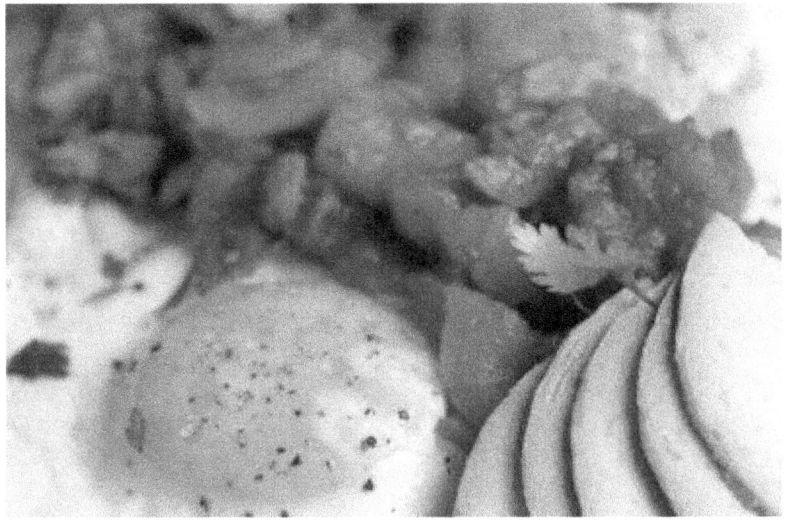

Serves 1

Ingredients

- ½ bell pepper, cut up nice and finely
- 1 fresh jalapeño, cut up nice and finely
- 1 tablespoon coconut oil
- ½ mild onion, cut up nice and finely
- 1 teaspoon freshly picked parsley, cut up nice and finely
- Freshly picked cilantro, cut up nice and finely
- 2 garlic cloves, crushed
- 1 tomato, cut up nice and finely
- 2 eggs
- ½ avocado

Method

Set your stove to Medium. Place half of the coconut oil into a heavy-based frying pan and let it melt. Put the pepper, chili, onion and the garlic in the pan and fry until the onion softens. Stir in the tomatoes and cook for another five minutes or so. Remove and set to one side.

In a clean pan, heat the remaining coconut oil and fry the eggs until done to your liking. Garnish with cilantro and serve.

19. Pulled Pork Afelia

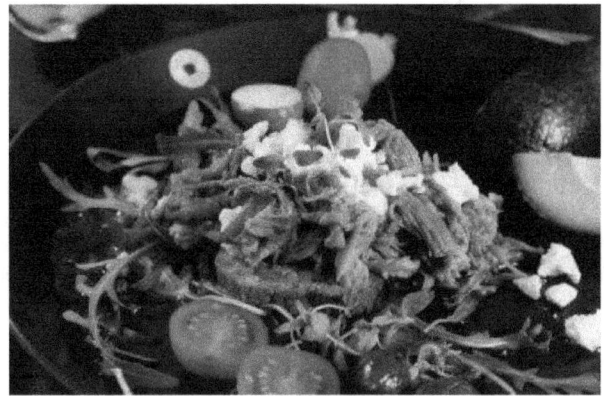

Serves 4

Ingredients

- 1 whole garlic bulb
- 2 red onions
- ¾ cup red wine
- 2 tablespoons coriander seeds, crushed
- 6¾ tablespoons olive oil
- 2 teaspoons dried thyme
- 2 teaspoons powdered cinnamon, powdered
- 2 teaspoons powdered black pepper
- 1 tablespoon salt
- 3⅓ pounds pork collars

Method

Peel the onions and slice them up into wedges. Peel the cloves and chop them into halves. Mix together all the other marinade ingredients and mix in half of the onion mixture. Clean the pork collar, pat it dry and then rub in salt to taste. Put it into the bag with the marinade. Make sure that the marinade is rubbed all over the meat. Get as much air out of the bag as possible and then seal it. Put in the refrigerator for a minimum of 12 hours.

Set your oven at 260. Grease an ovenproof dish and put the meat, along with the remaining onion mixture, into it in a single layer. Make sure you choose a dish that has a lid that fits on it snugly. Place in the oven and cook for between 5 and 6 hours or until the meat is done. Alternatively, you can cook it in the slow cooker on low for 10 hours.

20. Traditional Roast Chicken

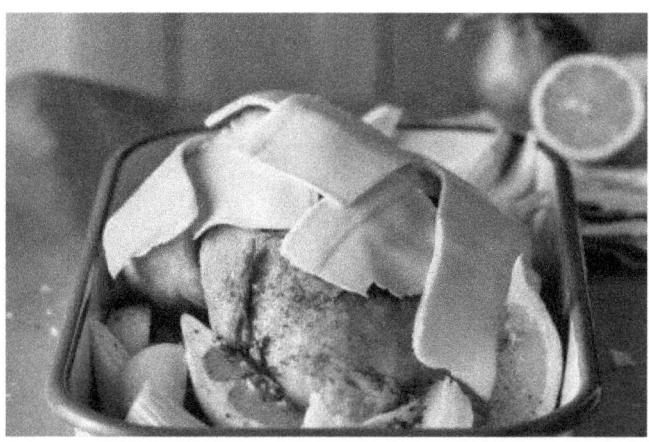

Serves 4

Ingredients

- Seasoning to taste
- 1 large chicken
- 3⅓ tablespoons water
- 2 teaspoons barbecue seasoning
- 1 lemon, cut into wedges
- ⅓ pound farm butter
- 2 mild onions

Method

Dry the chicken on the outside. Mix together salt and the barbeque seasoning. Grease a roasting tin and place the chicken into it. Chop the onions into evenly-sized wedges. Keep one wedge for the cavity of the chicken. Put the rest into the roasting dish. Do the same for the lemon. Cut the butter into thin slices and put it on top of the chicken.

Set your oven to 350. Put the chicken in the middle of the oven and cook for about 1½ hours. (Adjust the cooking time according to the size of your chicken.)

21. Oxtail

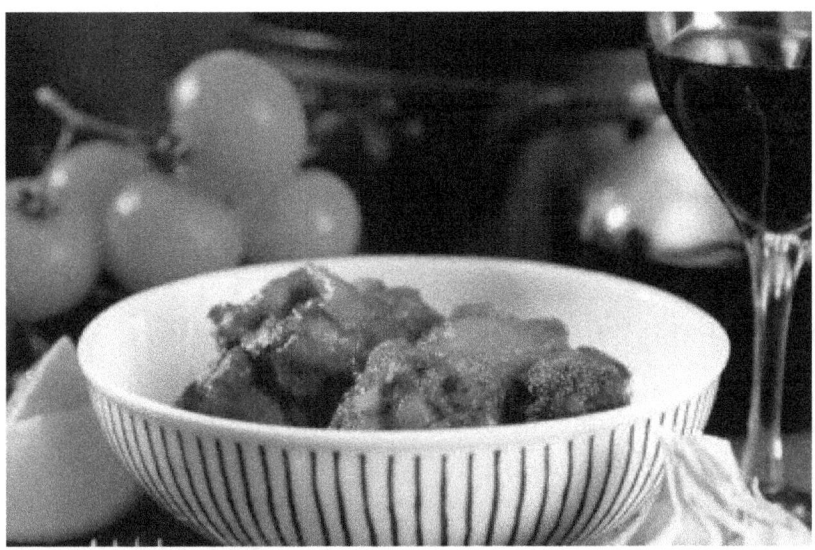

Serves 4

Ingredients

- 3 garlic cloves
- 8 pearl onions
- 3⅓ tablespoons tomato paste
- 2 pounds oxtails, cut into pieces
- Seasoning to taste
- 1¼ pound crushed tomatoes
- 1 orange
- powdered cinnamon sticks
- 2 tablespoons red wine vinegar
- ⅓ pound farm butter
- 2 bay leaf
- 1 tablespoon dried oregano

- 8 allspice berries
- 1 pinch ground cloves

Method

Peel the garlic and the onions and halve them. Set your stove to Med-High and melt the farm butter in a large frying pan. Cook the garlic and onions until the start to brown. Place them in a large pot. In the same pan, sear the meat and season as required. Put it into the large pot.

Grate off the zest of an orange into the large pot. Stir in the orange juice, the cinnamon, vinegar, tomatoes, allspice, bay leaves, cloves and oregano. Put 2 ounces of water into the frying pan, taking care to scrape all the leavings off the bottom.

Stir this in with the meat. Reduce the heat to Low and cook the meat for about 4 or 5 hours, stirring every now and again, until the meat is cooked through. You may need to also top up the water every now and again.

22. Lemon-Flavored Artichokes

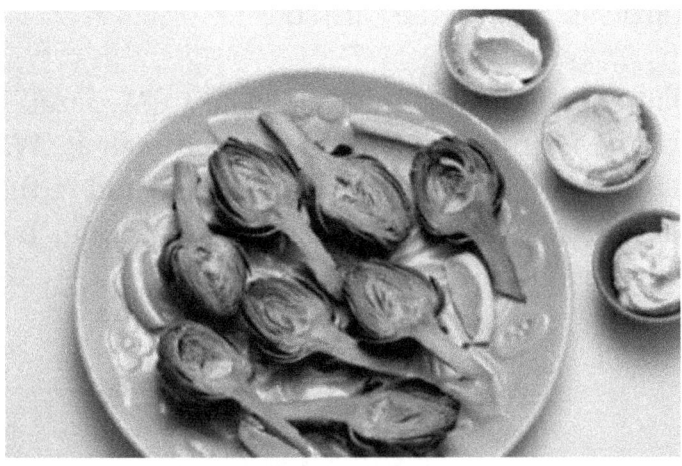

Serves 4

Ingredients

- 1 tablespoon salt
- ½ lemon
- 2 – 4 fresh artichokes

Ingredients for Lemon Farm Butter

- Seasoning to taste
- The juice and zest of ½ – 1 lemon
- 7 ounces of farm butter, cubed

Method

Remove the sharp edges of the artichokes. If you are using big artichokes, halve them before cooking. Set your stove to

Medium. Put the artichokes into a pot with enough water to cover them. Season to taste and then add half a fresh lemon. Boil the artichokes until they are soft.

While that is cooking, set another plate to Medium. Put two ounces of the farm butter unto a pot and melt it. Whisk the melted butter with the rest of the butter and add in the lemon juice. Season as required. The artichokes should be served warm with the butter as a dip.

23. Roasted Cauliflower and Onions

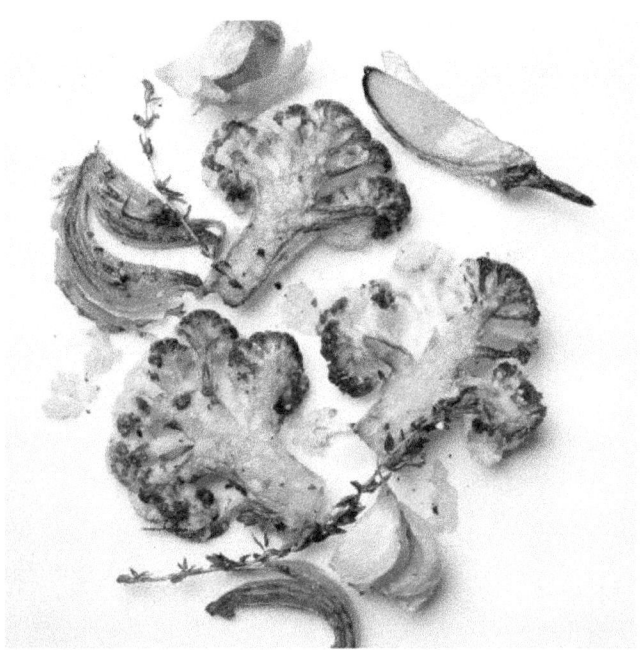

Serves 4

Ingredients

- Seasoning to taste
- ⅓ pound farm butter
- 2 pounds cauliflower
- 1 onion
- 2 sprigs of thyme

Method

Set your oven at 400. Chop the cauliflower into even-sized pieces. Chop the onion into wedges. Grease an oven-proof dish and put the cauliflower and onion on it in a single layer. Season as required. Dot with the farm butter. Top off with the sprigs of thyme. Put onto the uppermost rack of the oven and cook for about half an hour or until done.

24. Green Beans and Avocado

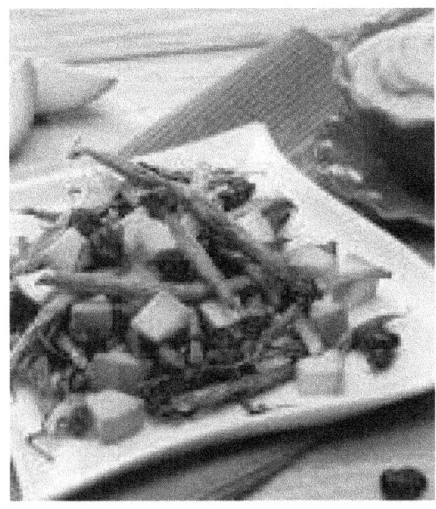

Serves 4

Ingredients

- ⅔ pound fresh green beans
- 3 tablespoons olive oil
- Freshly picked cilantro to taste
- ½ teaspoon table salt
- 2 ripe avocados
- ¼ teaspoon powdered black pepper
- 5 scallions

Method

Set your stove to Med-High. Warm up the oil in a large frying pan. Chop the scallions up nice and finely and put them in the pan, along with the beans. Stir-fry the beans and scallions until just done – about 4 or 5 minutes. Season to taste. Peel the avocado and cube it. Mix with the bean mixture and garnish with the cilantro.

25. Roasted Chicken with Creamy Béarnaise

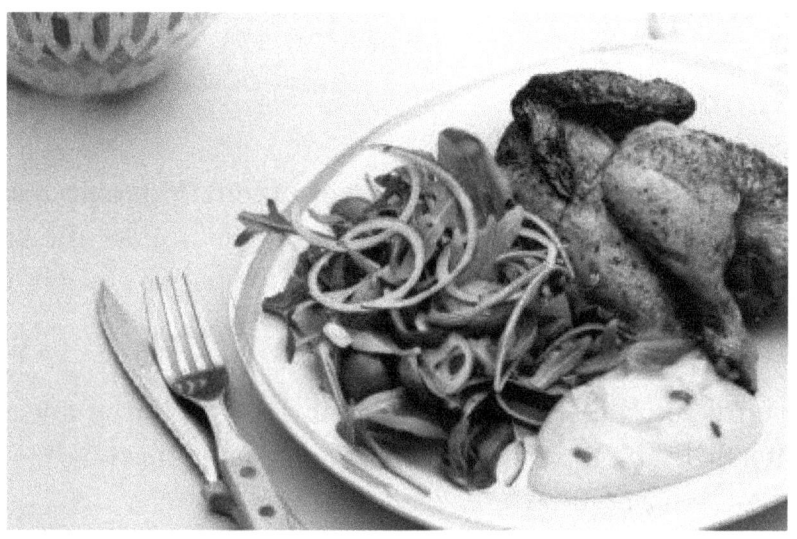

Serves 4

Ingredients

- Leafy greens
- 2 roasted chickens
- ½ a mild onion
- Pitted olives to taste

Ingredients for Spicy Béarnaise sauce

- 2 teaspoons white wine vinegar
- 4 egg yolks
- 2 pinches onion powder
- 2 teaspoons tomato paste

- 1 red chili pepper, deseeded and chopped up nice and finely
- 8¾ – 11 ounces of farm butter
- Seasoning to taste

Method

Cut the chickens into halves and plate them. Make up a salad using the greens, the onions and the olives. Make the sauce next. Put the egg yolks into a bowl and mix in the vinegar, chili and the onion powder.

Beat until completely combined. Melt the farm butter and then add it a little at a time to egg mixture, whisking thoroughly. Mix the tomato paste into the sauce and serve.

26. Lamb Sliders

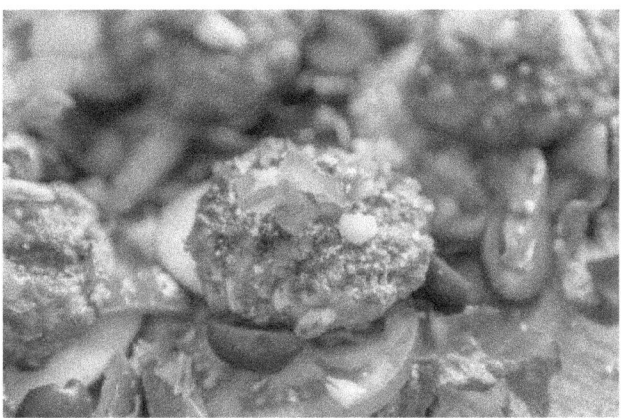

Serves 4

Ingredients

- ½ teaspoon table salt
- 1 pound ground lamb
- ½ teaspoon powdered black pepper
- The zest of 1 lemon
- 2 garlic cloves, crushed
- ¼ mild onion, chopped up nice and finely
- 2 teaspoons freshly picked oregano, chopped up nice and finely

Method

Season the lamb to taste. Mix in the onion, lemon zest, oregano and the onion. Divide the mixture into 8 equally sized balls and flatten into patties. Set your oven to Grill on Med-High. Grill the burgers for about 5 minutes per side.

27. Roasted Cabbage

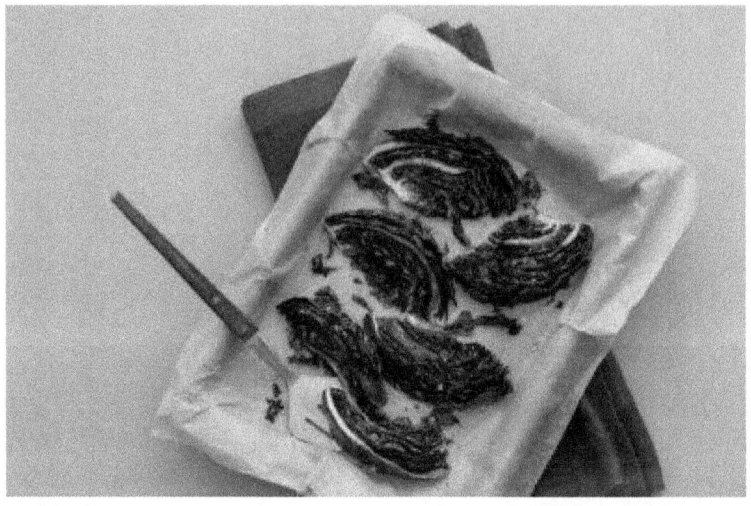

Serves 2

Ingredients

- 3 tablespoons olive oil
- 1 pinch powdered black pepper
- 1 pound red cabbage
- ½ teaspoon table salt

Method

Set your oven at 400. Take the core out of the cabbage and discard it. Chop the rest of the cabbage into thick wedges. Grease an oven-proof dish and line it with baking paper. Put the cabbage in the dish in a single layer. Season as you like and put the olive oil over the top. Put in the oven for about 25-30 minutes or until the cabbage is done throughout.

28. Endives to Die For

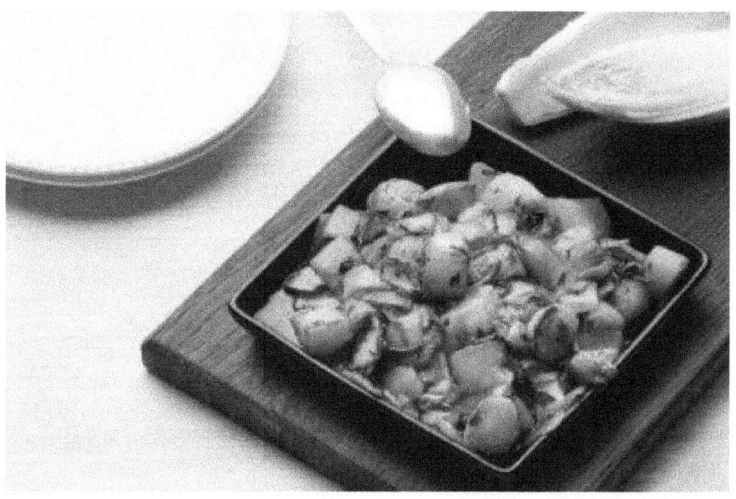

Serves 4

Ingredients

- 4¼ ounces of farm butter
- 2 pounds endives
- ½ teaspoon table salt
- 1 tablespoon freshly picked chives, chopped up nice & finely
- ¼ teaspoon powdered black pepper

Method

Set your stove to High. Melt the farm butter in a big heavy-based pan. Chop up the endives nice and finely and mix into the butter. Reduce the heat to Low until they are cooked through and nicely caramelized.

29. Spicy Scallops

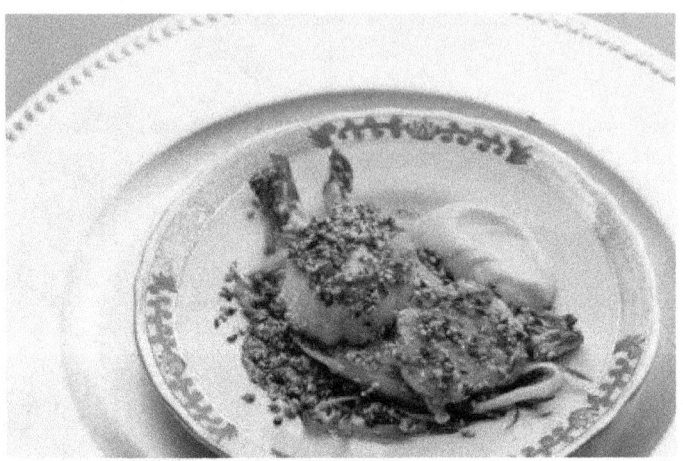

Serves 4

Ingredients

- 4 tablespoons Sesame seeds
- 8 scallops
- 1 tablespoon coconut oil
- 1 tablespoon lime juice
- ½ tablespoon wasabi paste
- 2 scallions
- 5⅓ tablespoons mayo
- 4 ounces of Bok Choy
- 1 tablespoon sesame oil

Method

Mix together the Wasabi paste, the mayo and the lime juice. Place the sesame seeds onto a side plate and coat the scallops with them. Set your stove to High. Grease a pan and cook the scallops for about half a minute on each side. Remove from the pan and set aside.

Chop the scallions nice and finely and do the same with the Bok Choy. Add the sesame oil to the pan and fry the scallions and the Bok Choy. Top off the greens with the scallops and serve.

I hope you have learned something from this book so far and would greatly appreciate it if you could leave an honest review on Amazon.com.

30. Buttered Scallops

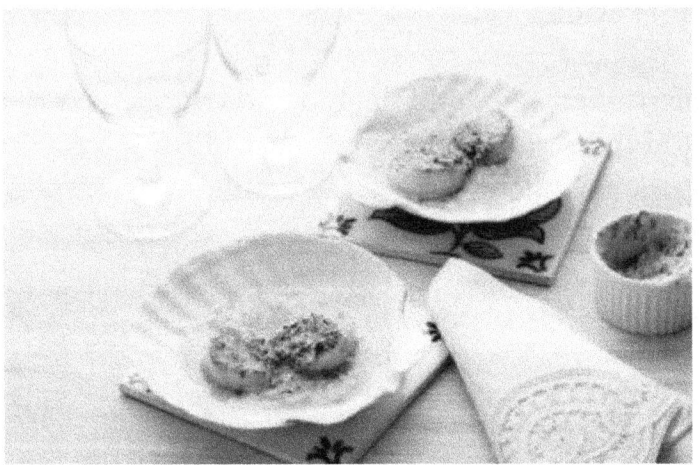

Serves 4

Ingredients

- 4¼ ounces of herb farm butter
- 8 scallops

Ingredients for Herb Farm Butter

- 2 garlic cloves
- 4¼ ounces of farm butter, softened
- ¼ teaspoon powdered black pepper
- 1 teaspoon lemon juice
- 2 tablespoons chopped freshly picked parsley
- 1 teaspoon table salt

Method

Set the stove to 450. Mix the ingredients for the herbed farm butter together and put to one side. Set the stove to high. Grease a frying pan and cook the scallops quickly for about 30 seconds per side. Put the scallops in ramekins and top them with the herbed farm butter. Put in the oven long enough to melt the butter and serve.

31. Scallops and Mash

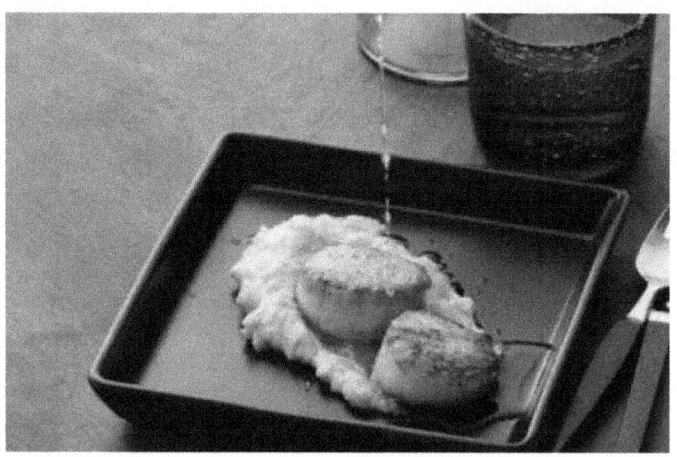

Serves 4

Ingredients

- Seasoning to taste
- 4¼ ounces of farm butter
- 8 scallops

Ingredients for the Mash

- Seasoning to taste
- 8 tablespoons water
- ⅓ pound parsnips
- 3¼ ounces of farm butter
- 1 teaspoon fennel seeds
- 1 teaspoon white wine vinegar

Method

Clean and peel all of the parsnips. Grate or chop them into fine pieces. Set your stove to Med-High. Put the parsnips in a pot and put in enough water to cover them. Add in 4 ounces of the butter.

Bring the water to the boil and cook for about 5 minutes. Reduce the heat to Low and cook until the parsnips soften up and most of the water has cooked away.

Mix in the vinegar and the spices and blend the parsnips until they have a smooth texture. Set the stove to High and melt the remaining butter in a frying pan. Fry the scallops in the butter for about 30 seconds per side. Serve on top of the parsnip mash.

32. Mussel Chowder

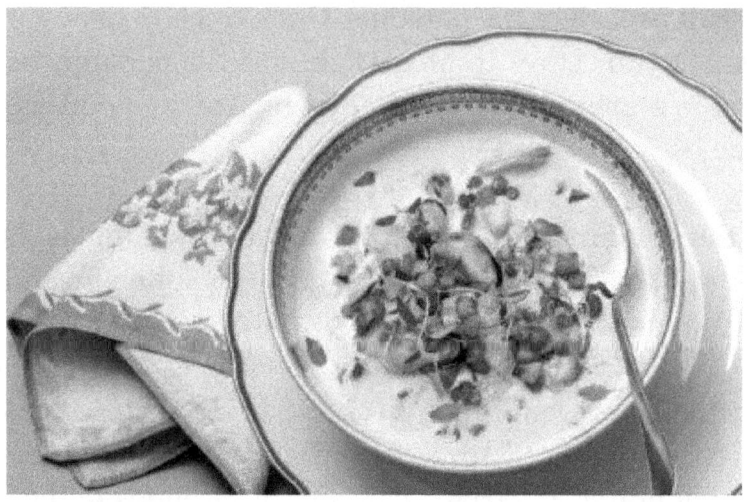

Serves 4

Ingredients

- ⅓ pound bacon
- 2 tablespoons farm butter
- 2 garlic cloves, chopped up nice and finely
- ½ pound root celery, diced
- 1 mild onion, chopped up nice and finely
- 1 cup of plain
- 2 cups double cream
- 1 tablespoon white wine vinegar
- 1 tablespoon freshly picked thyme, chopped up nice and finely
- 1 fish bouillon cube
- 1 bay leaf
- 2 cans mussels or clams

- Freshly picked thyme to use as a garnish
- Seasoning to taste

Method

Peel the onion and the garlic and chop them up nice and finely. Peel the root celery and cube it. Set the stove to High. Melt the farm butter in a heavy-based frying pan and fry the bacon until it crisps up. Take the bacon out of the pan and put to one side. Using the same pan, fry the veggies until they start to brown.

Add in the remaining ingredients, aside from the mussels. Let the mixture come to a boil. Reduce the heat to Low and allow it to simmer for another 10 minutes. Add the mussels and allow it to simmer for another few minutes. Garnish with the bacon and herbs.

33. Indian Stew

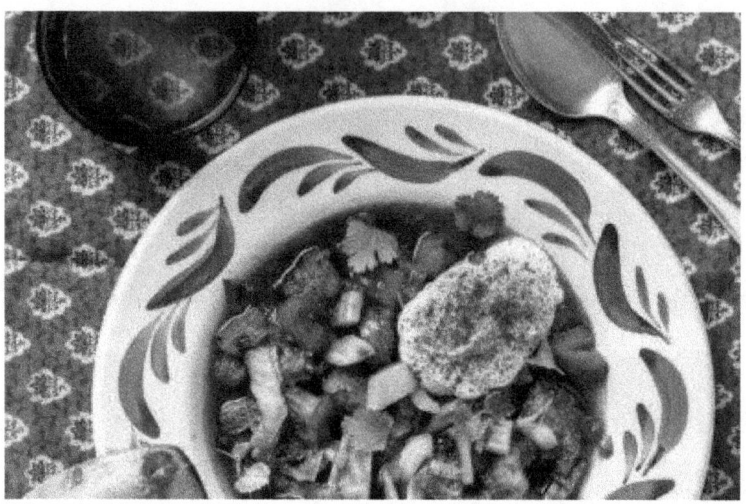

Serves 6

Ingredients

- 3 mild onions, chopped up nice and finely
- 2 pounds lamb shoulder, cut into bite-sized pieces
- 1 carrot, chopped up nice and finely
- 1 red chili, chopped up nice and finely
- 2 – 3 celery stalks
- 1 – 2 tablespoons curry powder
- 2 garlic cloves, chopped up nice and finely
- 1¾ ounces of farm butter
- 1 teaspoon table salt
- 1 can crushed tomatoes
- 1 lamb marrow bone
- 3⅓ tablespoons water

Serving

- 2 sliced bell peppers
- 6¾ tablespoons sour cream
- 2 Bok Choy, split into halves
- Fresh cilantro, chopped up nice and finely
- ½ leek, chopped up nice and finely

Method

This works really well in a tagine but if you don't have one, an oven-proof dish will work as well. Put the meat and the vegetables in the container. Put the marrow bone in the center of the dish.

Melt the farm butter and mix it with the curry and other spices. Drizzle over the dish. Add the water and the tomatoes. Put the dish into an oven set at 350. Cook for two or three hours or until the lamb is done.

Before serving, take the marrow bone out. If there is any marrow left in it, scoop it out. Mix in with the rest of the food and serve.

34. Roasted Lamb and Broccoli Mash

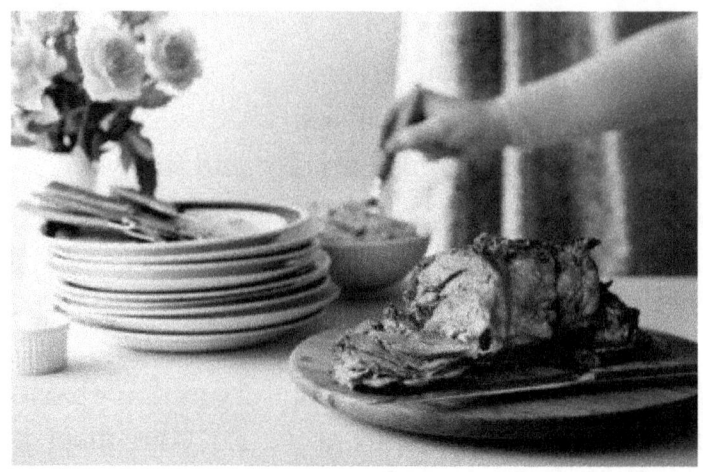

Serves 8

Ingredients for Lamb Roast

- Cooking string
- Seasoning to taste
- 3 pounds lamb roast
- 3 tablespoons freshly picked oregano, chopped up nice and finely
- 4¼ ounces of cream cheese
- The zest of ½ lemon
- 3 – 4 garlic cloves
- 3¼ ounces of farm butter

Ingredients for Broccoli Mash

- 2 pounds broccoli
- ⅔ pound Jerusalem artichokes

- ½ teaspoon powdered black pepper
- 1 teaspoon table salt
- 4¼ ounces of farm butter

Method

Set your oven to 320. Put the lamb with the skin side facing down. Season the roast to taste. Spread the cream cheese all over the inside of the roast. Sprinkle the garlic, lemon zest and herbs over the inside of the roast. Roll up and tie closed. Season the outside of the roast as required.

Grease a roasting tin and put the roast into it. Cook for at least an hour, the cooking time will depend on the actual weight of your roast. The roast is done when the internal temperature at the thickest part reaches 140. Allow the meat to rest for ten minutes before serving it.

Broccoli Mash: While the meat is cooking, peel the artichokes and chop them up nice and finely. Put them into a pot of water that has been seasoned. When the water comes to a boil, you should cook the artichokes for five minutes. Chop up the broccoli and add them to artichokes on the stove. Cook until they are both done. Drain well and mix in the farm butter. Adjust the seasoning if necessary and blend until smooth.

35. Delicate Fish Soup and Aioli

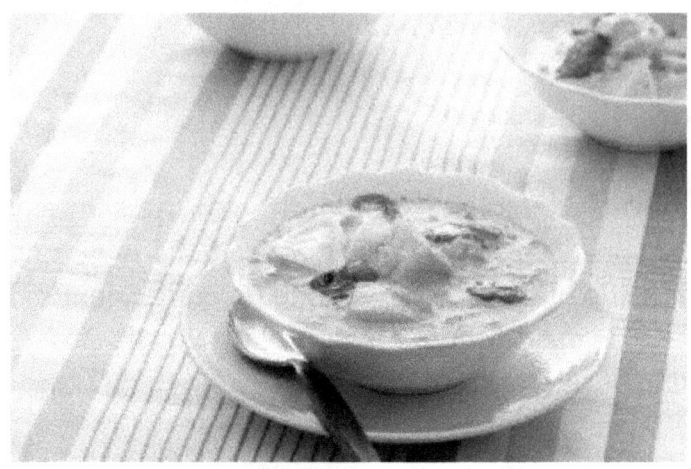

Serves 4

Ingredients

- 2 garlic cloves, chopped up nice and finely
- 1 mild onion, chopped up nice and finely
- ½ tablespoon tomato paste
- 1 fresh fennel
- 1 pinch saffron
- 2 fish bouillon cubes
- 2 cups water
- 1¼ cups sour cream
- Seasoning to taste
- 1 lime, the juice
- 8 cherry tomatoes
- freshly picked parsley, chopped up nice and finely
- 1½ pounds bite sized pieces of white fish

Ingredients for Aioli

- 1 tablespoon freshly picked parsley, chopped
- 1 – 2 garlic cloves, minced
- ½ – ⅗ cup mayo

Method

Set your stove to Medium. Fry together the garlic, onion, saffron and garlic in a little bit of water until they are soft. Stir the tomato paste in. Chop the tomatoes into quarters and put in the pot. Fry everything for another two or three minutes. Let the mixture come to a boil. Adjust seasoning as necessary. Reduce the heat to Low and cook for a further 10 minutes so that it can thicken.

Stir in the sour cream and the lime juice. Cook until the mixture boils and then add the fish. Simmer the soup for around 10 minutes or until the fish is cooked through. Garnish with the parsley just before you serve it. While that is cooking, mix the ingredients for the mayo together and serve with the soup.

Chapter 4

Snacks

1. Naan Bread

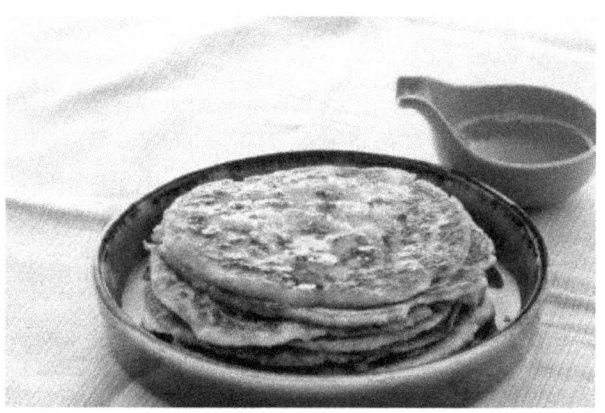

Servings 4

Ingredients

- ½ teaspoon baking powder
- 2 tablespoons powdered psyllium husks
- 1 teaspoon table salt
- table salt
- 2 cups boiling water
- 6¾ tablespoons coconut oil, melted
- coconut oil to fry the food in
- Garlic farm butter
- 1 – 2 garlic cloves, crushed
- 3½ ounces of farm butter

Method

Mix together the dry ingredients. Mix in the oil and the boiling water. Mix well and set aside for around 5 minutes to allow it to thicken up a little. It should be similar to Play-Doh in texture. Divide the dough into 8 evenly-sized balls. Flatten the balls out so that they are about half an inch thick.

Set your stove to Medium. Grease a frying pan with coconut oil and fry the bread until it is golden and done throughout. Set aside where it will be able to stay warm. Melt your farm butter, and stir in the garlic. Brush the butter on the Naan bread and season with salt. Use what is leftover as a dipping sauce.

2. Camembert Cheese Bake

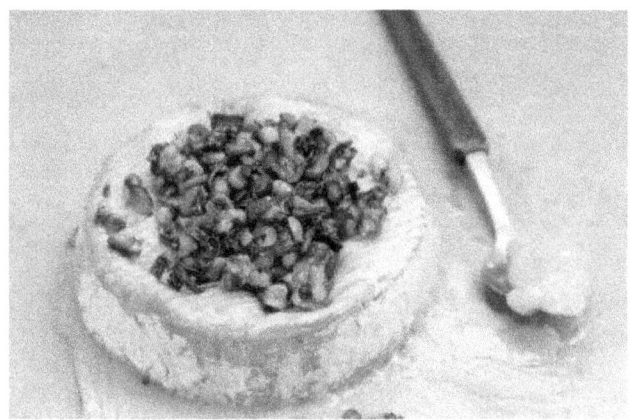

Servings 2

Ingredients

- 2 ounces of pecan nuts
- 8¾ ounces of Camembert cheese
- 1 garlic clove
- 1 tablespoon olive oil
- 1 tablespoon freshly picked thyme, chopped up nice and finely
- Seasoning to taste

Method

Set your oven at 400. Line a baking sheet with baking paper. Crush the garlic and chop up the nuts. Mix together with the olive oil and herbs. Top the cheese with it and put everything in the oven. Cook for around 10 minutes or till the cheese softens. Serve straight away.

3. Low-Carb Crispbread

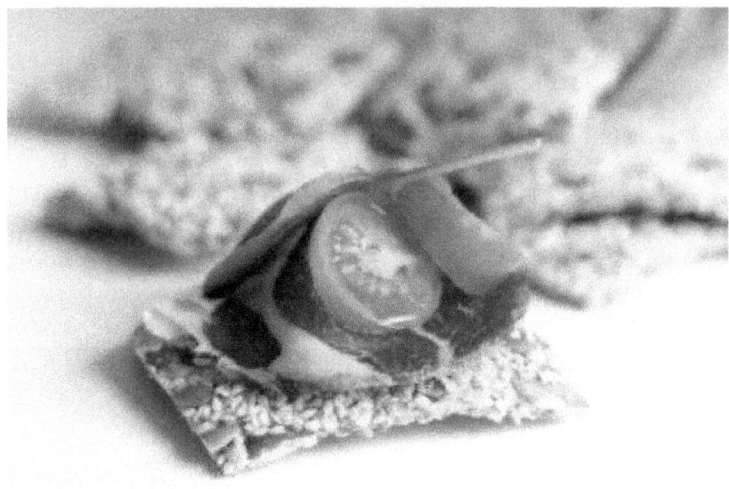

Serves 4

Ingredients

- 6¾ tablespoons sunflower seeds
- 1¼ cups Sesame seeds
- 2 ounces of Cheddar, grated
- 6¾ tablespoons water
- 1 tablespoon powdered psyllium husks
- 2 eggs
- Seasoning to taste

Method

Set your oven at 340. Mix all of the ingredients together. Line a baking tin with baking paper and spread the mixture out in a single layer. Season as required. Cook for around 20 minutes.

Remove from the oven and reduce the temperature to 280. Cut the mixture into pieces. Put it back in the oven and cook for about 40 minutes, or until completely dried out. Serve when cool.

4. Blueberry Smoothie

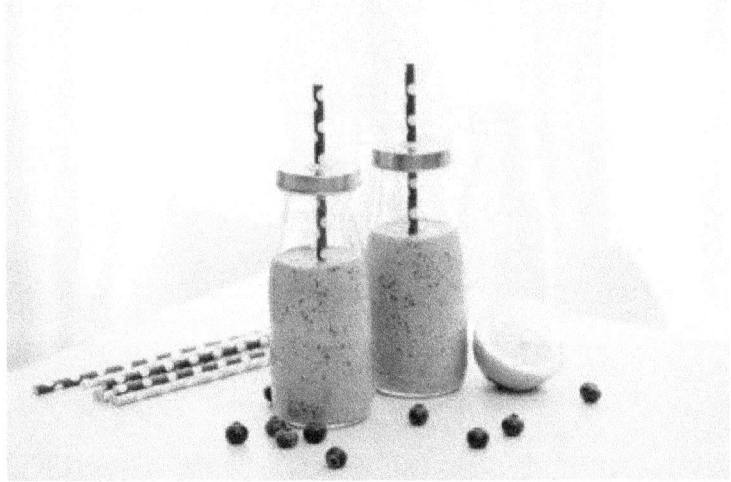

Serves 1

Ingredients

- ½ teaspoon vanilla essence
- 1 cup blueberries
- 1 2/3 cups coconut milk
- 1 tablespoon lemon juice

Method

Blend all of the ingredients together and serve straight away.

5. Strawberry Smoothie

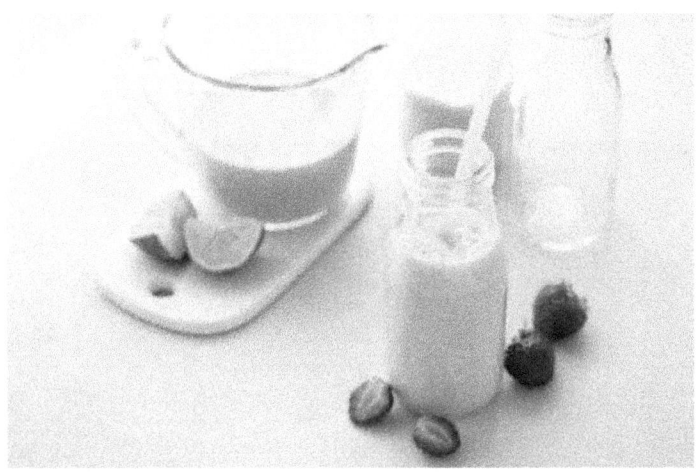

Serves 1

Ingredients

- ½ teaspoon vanilla essence
- 1 cup fresh strawberries
- 1 2/3 cups coconut milk
- 1 tablespoon lime juice

Method

Blend all of the ingredients together and serve straight away.

6. Low-Carb Buns

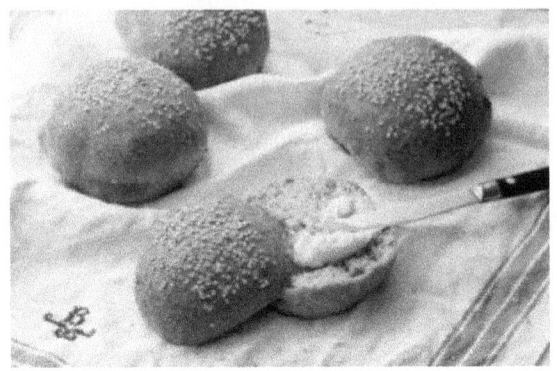

Serves 2

Ingredients

- 5 tablespoons powdered psyllium husks
- 1¼ cups almond flour
- 2 teaspoons baking powder
- 2 teaspoons apple cider vinegar
- 1 teaspoon table salt
- 1¼ cups boiling water
- Sesame seeds
- 3 egg whites

Method

Set your oven at 350. Mix together all the dry ingredients. Boil the water and stir into the egg and vinegar. Mix with the dry ingredients, ensuring that the dough is mixed well. Divide the mixture into 4 evenly-sized balls.

Grease a baking sheet and lay out the buns on it. Put on one of the lower oven racks and cook for around an hour. The buns are done when they sound hollow when tapped.

7. Salsa Dip

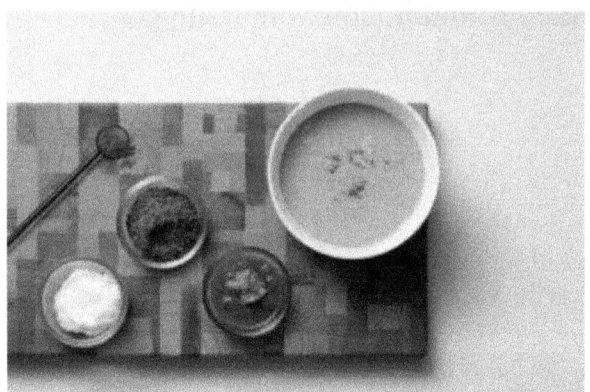

Serves 4

Ingredients

- 4 tablespoons extra virgin olive oil
- 1 garlic clove
- 8 tablespoons salsa sauce
- 2 tablespoons sour cream
- 3 tablespoons apple cider vinegar
- 2 tablespoons mayo
- 1 teaspoon chili powder

Method

Whisk everything together and season to taste.

8. Seed Crisps

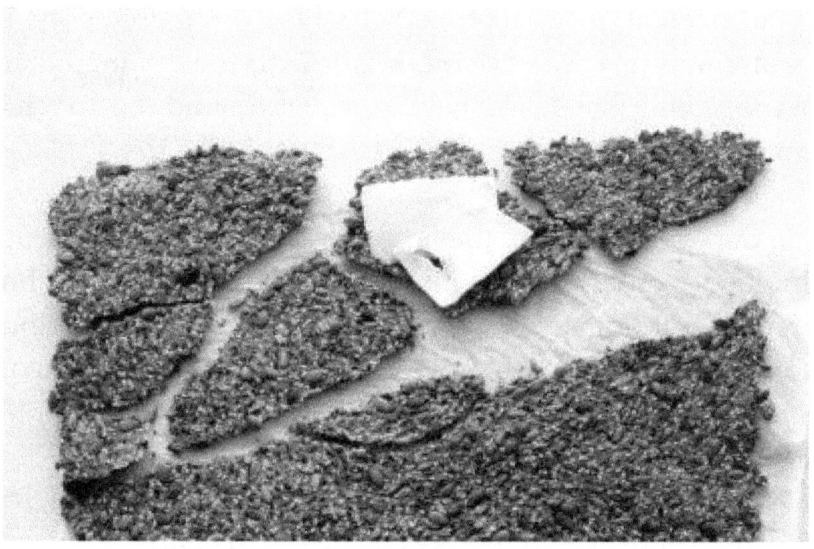

Serves 3

Ingredients

- 1 teaspoon table salt
- 5 1/3 tablespoons sunflower seeds
- 5 1/3 tablespoons almond flour
- 5 1/3 tablespoons pumpkin seeds
- 5 1/3 tablespoons Sesame seeds
- 5 1/3 tablespoons flax seeds
- 1 tablespoon powdered psyllium husks
- 4 tablespoons melted coconut oil
- Table salt
- 1 cup boiling water

Method

Set your oven at 300. Mix together all the dry ingredients. Boil the water and mix with the oil. Mix it with the dry ingredients. Line the baking sheet with baking paper. Spread the dough out into a thin and even layer. Sprinkle salt over the top.

Put in the oven on one of the bottom racks and cook for around 45 minutes or so. Do watch it to make sure that it doesn't burn. If they are not done, you need to bake for a further 15 minutes or so. Switch the oven off and leave the crisps in until the oven cools so that they can dry out more.

Don't forget to share your thoughts on this book by leaving a review on Amazon.com. It takes just a few seconds.

Are You ALWAYS Hungry When You Try to Lose Weight?

Discover How to STOP Starving Yourself & Lose Weight FASTER By Eating MORE Food!

For this month only, you can get Kayla's best-selling & most popular book absolutely free – *The Ultimate Guide to Healthy Eating & Losing Weight Without Starving Yourself!*

Get Your FREE Copy Here:
TopFitnessAdvice.com/Book

Discover how you can **start eating MORE food** and see weight loss results faster than ever before. Learn about the 10 most powerful fat-burning foods and how they boost the rate that your body burns fat. And last but not least, finally put an end to your emotional or "bored" eating habits. With this book, readers were able to significantly improve their weight loss results. So, it's highly recommended that you get this book, especially while it's free!

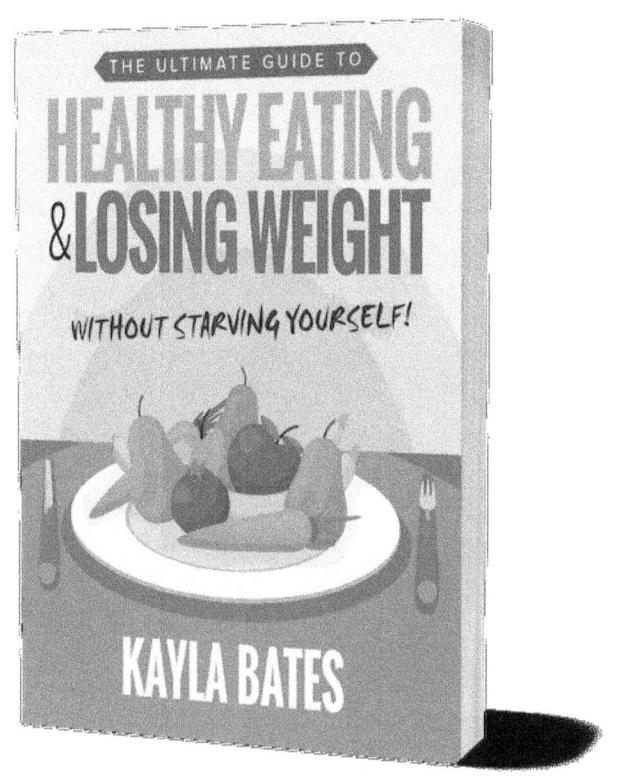

Get Your FREE Copy Here:
TopFitnessAdvice.com/Book

Conclusion

I hope that you have enjoyed these recipes and that you will have been inspired to try them out for yourself.

Once you understand something about how ketogenic recipes work, you can start to mix and match and experiment on your own.

With the great recipes in this book, you probably won't even feel like you are on diet. Losing weight could not be any easier.

Best of luck!

Enjoying this book?

Check out my other best sellers!

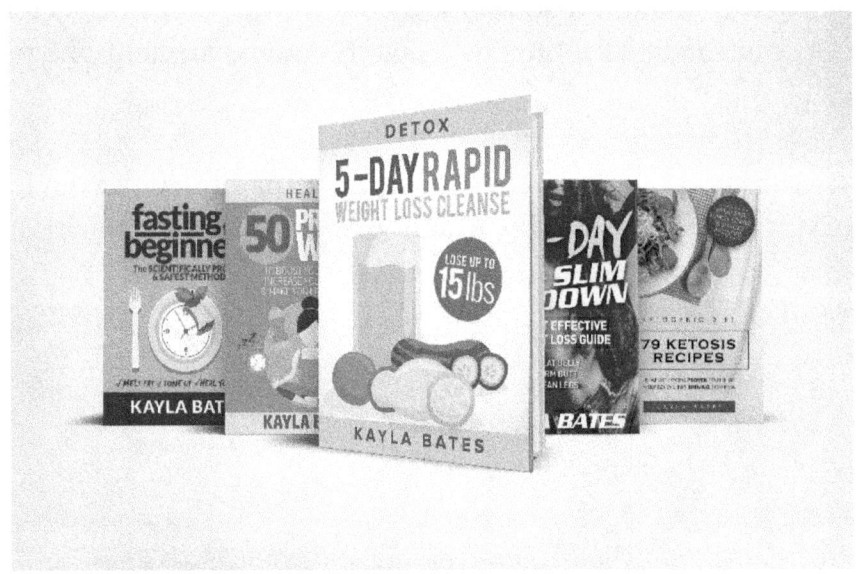

Get your next book on sale here:

TopFitnessAdvice.com/go/Kayla

Final Words

I would like to thank you for purchasing my book and I hope I have been able to help you and educate you on something new.

If you have enjoyed this book and would like to share your positive thoughts, could you please take 30 seconds of your time to go back and give me a review on my Amazon book page.

I greatly appreciate seeing these reviews because it helps me share my hard work.

You can leave me a review on Amazon.com.

Again, thank you and I wish you all the best!

www.ingramcontent.com/pod-product-compliance
Lightning Source LLC
Chambersburg PA
CBHW031154020426
42333CB00013B/654